Entry-Level
Respiratory Care Review

STUDY GUIDE
&
WORKBOOK

Entry-Level
Respiratory
Care Review

STUDY GUIDE
&
WORKBOOK

Second Edition

Gary Persing, BS, RRT
Director of Clinical Education
Respiratory Therapy Program
Tulsa Junior College
Tulsa, Oklahoma

W.B. SAUNDERS COMPANY
A Division of Harcourt Brace & Company
Philadelphia   London   Toronto   Montreal   Sydney   Tokyo

W.B. SAUNDERS COMPANY
A Division of Harcourt Brace & Company
The Curtis Center
Independence Square West
Philadelphia, PA 19106

For further information on Gary's Entry-Level Review Workshops, write to
Respiratory Review Workshops
1505 West Glendale Street
Broken Arrow, OK 74011
Or call:
(918) 455-0503

ENTRY-LEVEL RESPIRATORY CARE REVIEW: ISBN   0–7216–6426–1
STUDY GUIDE & WORKBOOK

Last digit is the print number: 9   8   7   6   5   4   3   2   1

*To my wonderful wife Debbie; my beautiful daughter Lindsey;
to my loving parents; and to God for His divine guidance.*

*This book is also dedicated to a very special group of
students who have made teaching an even greater experience
for me. Thanks for a fun two years.*

*1995 Therapist Graduates — Tulsa Junior College Respiratory
Therapy Program:*

Kerry Ashton
Mary Billings
Cynthia Carter
Brenda Duran
Bobbie Ford
Jimmie Howell
Melissa Kahler
John Moats
Mary Ojeda
Zoe Phillips
Kim Sigler
Robert Walker
Carla Wills
Woody Woodard

PREFACE

This combination study guide and workbook is a comprehensive review intended to prepare the student for the Entry-Level Certification Examination offered by the National Board for Respiratory Care (NBRC) and to become a Certified Respiratory Therapy Technician. The material covered in this book is based on the examination matrix provided by the NBRC. Because the NBRC examination excludes coverage of some of the most modern equipment, the clinical practices reflected in this book are not necessarily the most current in your region.

Each chapter in the Study Guide is preceded by Pretest questions. Before studying the chapter, answer these questions to test your present knowledge. The answers are at the end of each chapter. Then, begin reading the chapter carefully.

After completing the Study Guide, begin working with the Workbook. Answer all the questions you can without referring to the Study Guide. When you come to questions you can't answer, turn back to the corresponding roman numeral heading in the Study Guide. You will find the information needed to answer the question. Don't get discouraged if you find yourself frequently turning back and forth between the Study Guide and Workbook. By going back to the Study Guide and then answering the Workbook questions you will find a higher degree of retention of that material.

After completing each chapter in the Workbook, turn to the Posttest in the back of the Workbook. Find a quiet place and take this examination just as you would the real thing. The time limit is three hours, as it is for the Entry-Level Certification Examination. Grade the Posttest using the Answer Key immediately following the last page of the test. Pay close attention to areas in which you are weak and areas in which you are strong. After determining your weakest area, go back to the Study Guide and review.

You may also want to review the Workbook section. It is important to remember that the Study Guide section and Workbook section are to be used in conjunction with each other.

I conduct review workshops in various cities around the country, which many individuals have found to be beneficial in increasing their knowledge of entry-level material.

I feel strongly that with the use of this textbook, your previous educational experiences, your own abilities, and proper preparation you will soon be a Certified Respiratory Therapy Technician.

GARY PERSING
Tulsa, Oklahoma

CONTENTS

Study
Guide

Pulmonary Patient Assessment

PRETEST QUESTIONS*

1. A patient complains he has difficulty breathing while lying down. This condition is called

A. dyspnea.
B. orthopnea.
C. paroxysmal nocturnal dyspnea.
D. eupnea.

2. Which type of breath sound is heard over the entire chest wall except the supraclavicular area?

A. vesicular
B. bronchial
C. bronchovesicular
D. tracheal

3. A patient has a productive cough with expectoration of yellow sputum. What does this indicate about the patient's secretions?

I. They contain old blood.
II. A *Pseudomonas* infection is likely.
III. White blood cells are present in the sputum.
IV. The sputum is purulent.

A. I only
B. II and III only
C. III and IV only
D. I, III, and IV only

4. The type of breathing pattern characterized by deep, rapid breathing with progressively increasing and decreasing tidal volumes followed by an apneic episode is called

A. Biot's respiration.
B. Cheyne-Stokes respiration.
C. Kussmaul's respiration.
D. hyperventilation.

5. While palpating the chest of a patient, you notice that the trachea is shifted to the right and there is flatness to percussion on the right side. These findings are consistent with which of the following?

A. pneumothorax of the left lung
B. pulmonary embolus in the right lung
C. diffuse pulmonary emphysema
D. atelectasis of the right lung

6. In order to determine symmetrical chest movement of a patient, the respiratory care practitioner should do which of the following?

A. order a chest x-ray
B. have the patient lie supine and observe chest movement from the end of the bed
C. percuss the chest bilaterally
D. place a hand on the abdomen and observe abdominal movement

---

*See answers at the end of the chapter.

Pulmonary Patient Assessment

I. PATIENT HISTORY

A. Data to obtain from the patient
1. Chief complaint
2. Symptomatology — what symptoms the patient is exhibiting and when they started
3. Past medical problems
4. Occupation
5. Medications currently prescribed
6. Allergies
7. Patient's exercise tolerance and daily activities

II. ASSESSMENT OF SYMPTOMS

A. Common symptoms of pulmonary patients
1. **Cough** — aids in clearing the airway of secretions
   a. Nonproductive cough caused by the following:
      (1) Irritation of the airway
      (2) Acute inflammation of the respiratory mucosal membrane
      (3) Presence of a growth
      (4) Irritation of the pleura
      (5) Irritation of the tympanic membrane
   b. Productive cough — monitor sputum color
      (1) White and translucent — normal
      (2) Yellow — indicates infection and presence of white blood cells; termed **purulent**
      (3) Green — old, retained secretions
      (4) Green and foul smelling — *Pseudomonas* infection
      (5) Brown — old blood
      (6) Red — fresh blood
   c. When cough is productive, it is important to record the amount, consistency, odor, and color of sputum, as changes in these over a 24-hour period may be important in diagnosing pulmonary disease.
   d. Sputum collection and laboratory analysis are an important part of the pulmonary assessment. Steps in sputum collection include:
      (1) Explaining to patient the reason for collecting the sample
      (2) Maintaining good oral hygiene to prevent contamination by oral secretions
      (3) Ensuring that sputum is collected from a deep cough

NOTE: If patient cannot cough adequately, nasotracheal suctioning to obtain the sample may be necessary. To collect the sputum, a sputum trap or a Lukens tube catheter is necessary.

   e. Characteristics of a cough

(1) Barklike cough usually indicates croup.
(2) Harsh, dry cough with inspiratory stridor usually indicates upper airway problems.
(3) Wheezing-type coughs usually indicate lower airway pathology.
(4) Chronic productive coughs are indicative of chronic bronchitis.
(5) Frequent hacking cough and throat clearing may be the result of smoking or a sinus or viral infection.

2. **Dyspnea** — difficult or labored breathing
   a. A subjective symptom influenced by the patient's reactions and emotional state
   b. Causes of dyspnea
      (1) Increased airway resistance
      (2) Upper airway obstruction
      (3) Asthma and other chronic lung diseases
      (4) Decreased lung compliance
      (5) Pulmonary fibrosis
      (6) Pneumothorax
      (7) Pleural effusion
      (8) Abnormal chest wall
      (9) Anxiety state — no pathologic problem to explain it
   c. Types of dyspnea
      (1) **Orthopnea** — dyspnea while lying down. Usually a condition seen in patients with heart failure and chronic lung disease and results from increased congestion of the lungs while lying down or ineffective diaphragmatic breathing.
      (2) **Paroxysmal nocturnal dyspnea** — sudden onset of shortness of breath after being in bed several hours. Seen with cardiac patients and results in acute pulmonary edema that usually subsides quickly.
      (3) **Exertional dyspnea** — often observed in patients with cardiopulmonary disease. The severity is determined by the amount of exertion.

3. **Hemoptysis** — the coughing up of blood from the respiratory tract
   a. Blood-tinged or blood-streaked sputum is not termed hemoptysis.
   b. Hemoptysis is determined by the coughing up of certain volumes of blood. The amount of bleeding indicates the severity of the hemoptysis.
   c. Causes of hemoptysis
      (1) Pneumonia
      (2) Tuberculosis
      (3) Bronchiectasis
      (4) Lung abscess
      (5) Fungal lung infection — histoplasmosis
      (6) Neoplasms — bronchogenic carcinoma
      (7) Pulmonary embolism
      (8) Valvular heart diseases
      (9) Mitral valve stenosis
   d. The patient may report "coughing up blood" when the blood is actually from the stomach or elsewhere. The origin of the bleeding must be determined.

4. **Chest pain**
   a. The thoracic wall is the most common source of chest pain.
   b. The pain may be from nerves, muscles, skin, or bones of the thoracic wall.
   c. The lung parenchyma is not sensitive to pain.
   d. The parietal pleura (layer lining the chest wall) is very sensitive to pain and is usually responsible for the pain associated with pneumonias, pleurisy, and other inflammatory processes.
   e. Chest pain may be associated with pulmonary hypertension due to the increased tension on the walls of the vessels and increased work load on the right side of the heart.
   f. Chest pain may originate from the heart owing to inadequate blood supply. This pain is called **angina pectoris.**
   g. Chest pain is also associated with a ruptured aorta, myocardial infarction, and esophageal problems.

III. OTHER PHYSICAL ASSESSMENTS

A. **Breathing patterns**
1. **Eupnea** — normal rate and depth of respirations. Normal rate is 10 to 20 breaths per minute.
2. **Bradypnea** — lower than normal respiratory rate. May be seen with respiratory center depression due to head trauma or drug overdose.
3. **Apnea** — absence of breathing for a specific period of time (usually at least 10 seconds). Seen with respiratory arrest due to asphyxia, severe drug overdose, or **obstructive sleep apnea.**
4. **Tachypnea** — above-normal respiratory rate with a normal depth of breathing. May indicate decreased lung compliance and is associated with restrictive diseases, pneumonia, and pulmonary edema.
5. **Hypopnea** — shallow respirations (about half of normal depth) with slower-than-normal respiratory rate. Normal in well-conditioned athletes and accompanied by a slow pulse rate. May be seen with damage to the brainstem accompanied by a weak, rapid pulse.
6. **Hyperpnea** — deep, rapid, and labored breathing. Associated with conditions in which there is an inadequate oxygen supply, as in cardiac and respiratory diseases. Usually refers to hyperventilation.
7. **Kussmaul's respiration** — increased rate and depth of breathing. Usually seen in patients with severe metabolic acidosis (diabetic ketoacidosis).
8. **Biot's respiration** — irregular depth of breathing with periods of apnea. Breathing may be slow and deep or rapid and shallow. Associated with elevated intracranial pressure (ICP) or meningitis.
9. **Cheyne-Stokes respiration** — deep, rapid breathing followed by an apneic period. The breaths begin slow and shallow and gradually increase to above normal volume and rate, then gradually diminish in volume and rate followed by apnea. Apnea may last 10 to 20 seconds before the cycle is repeated. Seen with respiratory center depression due to stroke or head injury, pneumonia in the elderly, or drug overdose.

B. **Chest inspection** — should be performed with the patient seated and clothing removed above the waist. If unable to sit in a chair, the patient should be placed in bed in the Fowler's position (head of bed elevated 45°). **Inspection should include:**
1. Rate, depth, and regularity of breathing compared with norms for the patient's age and activity level
2. Skin color, temperature, and condition (e.g., bruises or scars). Is skin diaphoretic (perspiring)?
3. Chest symmetry — comparison of one side of the chest with the other.
   a. Observe chest excursion while standing in front of the patient or standing at the foot of the bed of a supine patient to determine if both sides are expanding equally.
   b. Unequal expansion may indicate:
      (1) Atelectasis
      (2) Pneumothorax
      (3) Chest deformities
      (4) Flail chest — paradoxical respirations in which chest moves in on inspiration and out on expiration
4. Shape and size of chest compared with normal
   a. Observe the anterior-posterior (A-P) diameter.
   b. An increased A-P diameter is called a **"barrel chest" and is indicative of chronic lung disease.**
5. Work of breathing
   a. Should be evaluated to determine the level of breathing difficulty
   b. While observing the patient's breathing process, determine the following factors:
      (1) Is chest movement symmetrical?
      (2) Are the accessory muscles being used?
      (3) What is the shape of the chest?
      (4) What is the respiratory rate?
      (5) Is the breathing pattern regular or irregular?
      (6) Are there any bony deformities of the ribs, spine, or chest?
      (7) Is the patient's tidal volume normal for size and age?
      (8) Is expiration prolonged, shorter than inspiration, or equal to inspiration?
      (9) Are substernal, suprasternal, or intercostal retractions or nasal flaring observed?

C. **Inspection of the extremities**
1. Digital clubbing

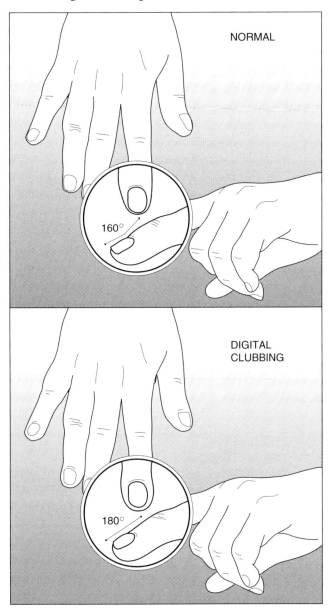

a. Digital clubbing is indicative of longstanding pulmonary disease (75 to 85% of all clubbing is the result of pulmonary disease).
b. It is an enlargement of the distal phalanges of the fingers and, less commonly, the toes. There is a loss of the angle between the nail and dorsum of the terminal phalanx.
c. It is the result of **chronic hypoxemia.**

2. Pedal edema
a. This refers to an accumulation of fluid in the subcutaneous tissues of the ankles.
b. This symptom is commonly observed in patients with chronic pulmonary disease, whose chronic hypoxemic state results in pulmonary vasoconstriction.
c. This results in an increased workload on the right heart, right ventricular hypertrophy, and eventually, right heart failure (cor pulmonale).
d. Venous blood flow returning to the heart is diminished, and the peripheral blood vessels become engorged. The ankles are most affected due to gravity dependency.

3. Cyanosis
a. This term refers to the bluish discoloration of the skin and nailbeds resulting from a 5 gm/dL decrease in oxygenated hemoglobin.
b. Cyanosis may indicate decreased oxygenation or reduced peripheral circulation.
c. Patients with decreased hemoglobin levels (anemia) may not exhibit cyanosis even if tissue hypoxia is present. An anemic patient has a low oxygen carrying capacity, which may result in tissue hypoxia, but will not be cyanotic unless 5 gm/dL of unsaturated hemoglobin is present, which may not be the case.
d. Conversely, a patient with an increased level of hemoglobin (polycythemia) has an increased capacity for carrying oxygen. This patient may have 5 gm/dL of unsaturated hemoglobin, and therefore be cyanotic, yet have enough saturated hemoglobin to adequately oxygenate the tissues.

4. Capillary refill
a. Perfusion to the extremities may be determined by assessing capillary refill.
b. This is performed by compressing the patient's fingernail for a short time, then releasing it and observing the time it takes for blood flow to return to the nailbed.
c. Normal refill time is less than three seconds.
d. Patients with decreased cardiac output and poor digital perfusion will have a longer refill time.

D. **Chest deformities**

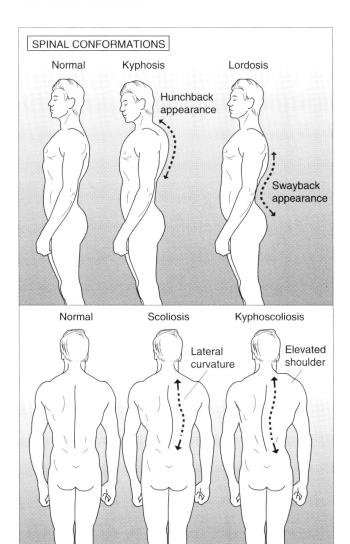

SPINAL CONFORMATIONS

Normal | Kyphosis | Lordosis

Hunchback appearance

Swayback appearance

Normal | Scoliosis | Kyphoscoliosis

Lateral curvature

Elevated shoulder

1. **Kyphosis**
   a. Backward curvature of the thoracic spine resulting in a "hunchback" appearance
   b. Caused by degenerative bone disease or age, or may be associated with chronic obstructive pulmonary disease (COPD)
2. **Lordosis**
   a. Backward curvature of the lumbar spine resulting in a "swayback" appearance
   b. Usually not responsible for respiratory difficulties
3. **Scoliosis**
   a. Lateral curvature of the thoracic spine resulting in posterior protrusion of the chest and flattening out of the anterior ribs
   b. Depending on severity, it may result in impaired lung movement.
4. **Kyphoscoliosis**
   a. Combination of kyphosis and scoliosis

b. May be best observed by noting different heights of the shoulders
   c. Cardiopulmonary problems do not normally present until patient reaches the age of 40 or 50.
   d. Pulmonary signs and symptoms of kyphoscoliosis
      (1) Dyspnea
      (2) Hypoxemia
      (3) Hypercapnia
      (4) Progressive respiratory insufficiency
      (5) Eventual cardiac failure
      (6) Decreased lung capacities evidenced on pulmonary function tests (**restrictive disease**)
      (7) Frequent pulmonary infections
      (8) Uneven ventilation-perfusion ratio

5. **Pectus carinatum**

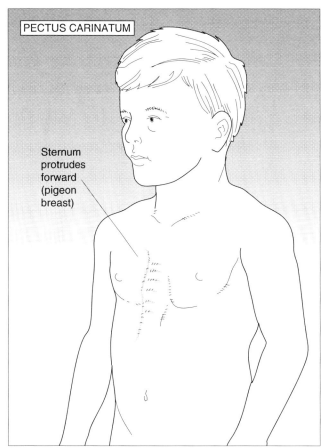

PECTUS CARINATUM

Sternum protrudes forward (pigeon breast)

a. Also called "pigeon breast" — results in forward projection of the xiphoid process and lower sternum
   b. Usually a congenital condition
   c. May cause dyspnea on exercise and more frequent respiratory infections due to interference with heart and lung movement
   d. In severe cases, surgical correction may be indicated.

6. **Pectus excavatum**

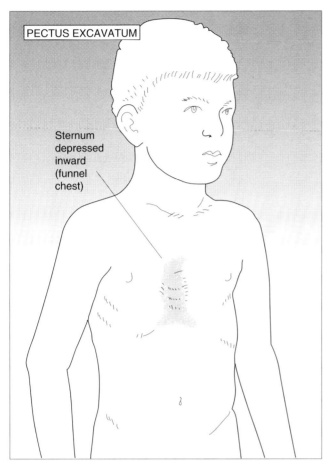

a. Also called "funnel chest" — results in a funnel-shaped depression over the lower sternum
b. Usually a congenital condition
c. May lead to dyspnea on exertion and more frequent respiratory infections
d. Reduces the ability to eat a full meal; therefore, many patients are underweight

7. **Barrel chest**

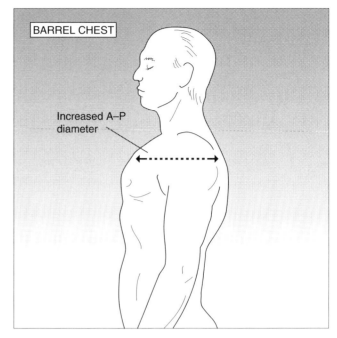

a. Caused by premature closure of the airways, resulting in air trapping and hyperinflated lungs that give the chest a barrel appearance
b. Also contributing is the increased musculature from the accessory muscles which are used during normal breathing by COPD patients. The accessory muscles include the sternomastoids, the scalenes, the abdominals, and the pectoralis major. These muscles are normally not used for quiet ventilation, but when ventilatory demand increases. Such is the case in the severe COPD patient with less than adequate diaphragmatic utilization.
c. Seen almost exclusively in patients with chronic lung disease.
d. This hyperinflated state of the lungs pushes down on the diaphragm, restricting its movement. This decreases alveolar ventilation and chest excursion, resulting in an increased work of breathing.
e. The diaphragm and external intercostals are the muscles normally used for ventilation. However, COPD patients have a flattened diaphragm and must use their accessory muscles during normal ventilation.

E. **Palpation of the chest**

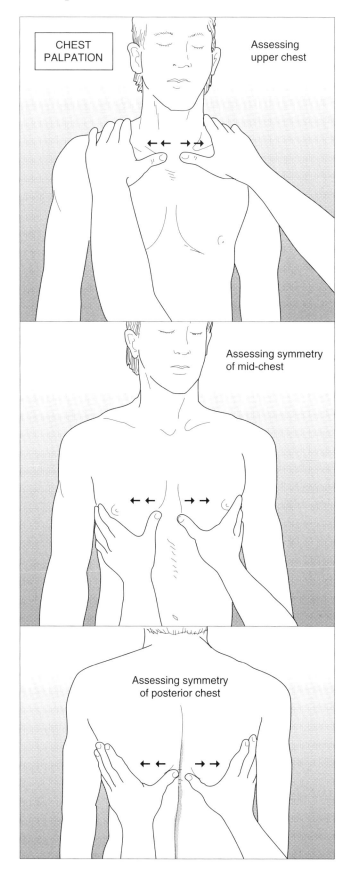

1. Using the sense of touch on the chest wall to assess physical signs
2. Hands are placed on the chest to assess chest movement and vibration.
3. Tactile fremitus (vibration)
   a. The patient is asked to say certain words (such as "ninety-nine") and the practitioner moves his/her hands to feel over different areas of the chest.
   b. Vibrations are decreased over areas of atelectasis, fluid, pneumothorax, or masses.
   c. Increased vibrations are heard with pneumonia.
4. Crepitus
   a. Crepitus is the term used to describe the feeling one gets when palpating the chest of a patient with an air leak present.
   b. Crepitus during chest palpation is indicative of subcutaneous emphysema caused by a pneumothorax.
5. Position of the trachea

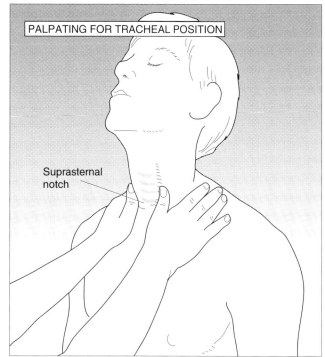

   a. Assessed by placing both thumbs on each side of the sternal notch and gently pressing inward. One should feel soft tissue only. If the trachea is felt, this indicates the trachea has shifted and is no longer positioned at the midline as it should be.
   b. A shift of the trachea may be the result of a pneumothorax or atelectasis.
      (1) In pneumothorax, **the trachea is shifted**

to the unaffected side (opposite side of pneumothorax)

(2) In atelectasis, **the trachea is shifted toward the affected side (same side as atelectasis)**

F. **Percussion of the chest wall**
1. Tapping on the chest directly with one finger or indirectly by placing one finger on chest area and tapping on that finger over different areas of the chest
2. There are five different sounds heard on percussion:
   a. Hyperresonance — recognized by a loud, low-pitched sound of long duration produced over areas that contain more air than tissue. Examples: air-filled stomach, emphysema (air trapping), pneumothorax
   b. Resonance — recognized by a low-pitched sound of long duration produced over areas with equal distribution of air and tissue. Example: normal lung tissue
   c. Dullness — recognized by a sound of medium intensity and pitch with a short duration produced over areas containing more tissue or fluid than air. Examples: atelectasis, consolidation, pleural effusion, pleural thickening, pulmonary edema
   d. Flatness — recognized by a sound of low amplitude and pitch produced over areas containing more tissue than air. Examples: massive pleural effusion, massive atelectasis, pneumonectomy
   e. Tympany — recognized by a "drumlike" sound. Example: tension pneumothorax
G. **Auscultation of breath sounds**
1. **Normal breath sounds**
   a. **Vesicular**
      (1) Gentle rustling sound heard over the entire chest wall except the right supraclavicular area
      (2) Inspiration is longer than expiration, with no pause between the two.
   b. **Bronchial**
      (1) Loud and generally high-pitched sound heard over the upper portion of the sternum, trachea, and main-stem bronchi
      (2) Expiration is longer than inspiration, with a short pause between the two.
      (3) If heard in other lung areas, indicative of atelectasis or consolidation
   c. **Bronchovesicular**
      (1) Combination of bronchial and vesicular

breath sounds normally heard over the sternum, between the scapulae, and over the right apex of the lung

(2) Inspiration and expiration are of equal duration, with no pause between the two.

   d. **Tracheal**
      (1) Harsh and high-pitched sound heard over the trachea
      (2) Expiration is slightly longer than inspiration.
2. **Adventitious breath sounds**
   a. **Rales (crackles)**
      (1) Bubbling or crackling sound heard primarily on inspiration, produced by air flowing through fluid in the alveoli or small airways
      (2) **Rales** are commonly heard when pulmonary edema, pneumonia, or emphysema is present.
   b. **Rhonchi**
      (1) Sounds produced in airways filled with secretions or fluids. They have a typical rumbling sound and are heard on expiration.
      (2) Heard primarily in larger airways
      (3) Caused by asthma, emphysema, mucous plugs, or stenosis

NOTE: A distinguishing feature between rales and rhonchi is that rhonchi will generally clear after coughing, while rales usually will not.

   c. **Wheezes**
      (1) Often considered rhonchi with a musical quality and produced by air flowing through constricted airways
      (2) May be heard on both inspiration and expiration
      (3) Wheezes are characteristically heard with asthma due to bronchoconstriction.
   d. **Pleural friction rub**
      (1) A clicking or grating sound caused by friction produced as the parietal and visceral pleurae rub against each other during breathing
      (2) Most commonly associated with pleurisy and is very painful
H. **Chest x-ray interpretation**
1. Useful terms when interpreting chest x-rays
   a. **Anterior-posterior (A-P)** — chest x-ray taken from front to back
   b. **Consolidation** — well-defined, solid-

appearing lung. Appears light on x-ray. **Caused by pneumonia**

c. **Radiodensity** — descriptive of white areas on the x-ray. Fluids and solids appear white. **Caused by pneumonia, bony areas, and pleural effusion**

d. **Infiltrates** — scattered or patchy white areas on x-ray. Due to inflammatory processes. **Caused by atelectasis or disease processes**

e. **Radiolucency** — appears dark on x-ray. Air is dark on x-ray. Hyperlucency (excessive darkness on x-ray) is characteristic of emphysema, asthma, or subcutaneous emphysema.

2. Respiratory care practitioners most commonly observe chest x-rays for the following:

a. **Atelectasis**
   (1) Appears lighter than normal lung tissue
   (2) Elevated diaphragm, mediastinal shift (toward area of atelectasis), increased density, and decreased volume of lung area may be observed.

b. **Pneumonia**
   (1) Appears white on x-ray
   (2) Consolidation of entire lobe or more, causing **mediastinal shift toward the consolidation**

c. **Pneumothorax**
   (1) Air found in the pleural cavity, appearing dark with no vascular markings in the involved areas.
   (2) **Tension pneumothorax** may result in mediastinal shift, and a shift of the trachea **away from the side of the pneumothorax may be observed.**

d. **Endotracheal (E-T) tube placement**
   (1) End of tube should rest 2 to 7 cm above the carina.
   (2) Carina is located on x-ray at the level of the fourth rib or fourth thoracic vertebra.
   (3) If E-T tube is inserted too far, it has a greater tendency to enter the **right main-stem bronchus.**
   (4) If right main-stem is inadvertently intubated, diminished breath sounds may be heard on the left, and asymmetrical chest movement is possible with the right side expanding more than the left.

e. **Heart shadow**
   (1) Heart should appear white in the middle of the chest, with the left border easily determined

   (2) A normal heart should be less than half the width of the chest. Increased heart size may indicate congestive heart failure.

f. **Diaphragm**
   (1) Should be rounded or dome-shaped
   (2) Appears white on x-ray at the level of the sixth rib
   (3) Patients with hyperinflated lungs (COPD) will have a flattened diaphragm.
   (4) Both hemidiaphragms should be assessed for height and angle to the chest wall.
   (5) The dome of the right hemidiaphragm is normally 1 to 2 cm higher than the left because of the position of the liver.
   (6) Elevation of one hemidiaphragm may be the result of gas in the stomach or lung collapse.

I. **Pulse**
   1. Pulse is a direct indicator of heart action.
   2. Normal heart rate in adult: 60 to 90 beats/min
   3. Normal heart rate in child: 90 to 120 beats/min
   4. An abnormally low heart rate is called **bradycardia.** Caused by infection, hypothermia, and heart abnormalities.
   5. An abnormally high heart rate is called **tachycardia.** Caused by hypoxemia, fever, loss of blood volume, heart abnormalities, and anxiety.
   6. Peripheral edema may indicate inadequate pumping action of the heart resulting from right heart failure (cor pulmonale).

J. **Blood pressure** — measured with a **sphygmomanometer**
   1. A measurement of the pressure within the arterial system
   2. Normal range for adults: 100 to 140/60 to 90 mm Hg
   3. Normal range for children: varies depending on age
   4. Normal range for neonates: 60 to 90/30 to 60 mm Hg
   5. Systolic (top number) pressure is the pressure measured during ventricular contraction.
   6. Diastolic (bottom number) is the pressure measured while the ventricles are at rest.
   7. The diastolic pressure is the most critical measurement, as it is the lowest pressure that the heart and arterial system will be subjected to.
   8. An abnormally low blood pressure is called **hypotension.** Caused by shock, volume loss, positioning, and depressant drugs.

9. An abnormally high blood pressure is called **hypertension**. Caused by cardiovascular imbalances, stimulant drugs, stress, and fluid retention due to renal failure.
10. Factors that affect blood pressure:
    a. Blood volume
    b. Blood viscosity
    c. Heart's pumping action
    d. Elasticity of blood vessels
    e. Resistance to blood flow through the vessels

K. **Body temperature**
   1. Normal body temperature is 98.6°F or 37°C. Temperature is slightly higher in children owing to higher metabolic rate.
   2. An abnormally low body temperature is called **hypothermia**. Caused by sweating (diaphoresis), blood loss, exposure, and increased heat loss.
   3. An abnormally high body temperature is called **hyperthermia**. Caused by decreased heat loss, infection, or increased environmental temperature.
   4. The term used for a condition of normal body temperature is **afebrile** (literally, "without fever").

L. **Assessing mental status**
   1. **Level of consciousness**
      a. Alert — patient is awake and responds to stimuli
      b. Obtunded and confused — patient is awake but responds slowly to commands; may be disoriented
      c. Lethargic — patient seems unconscious but will awaken when stimulated
      d. Coma — patient is unconscious and will not awaken when stimulated
   2. **Orientation to time and place**
      a. Ask patient the date.
      b. Ask patient where he/she is.
   3. **Ability to cooperate**
      a. Ask patient to follow simple commands.
      b. Must have patient cooperation for effective therapy, such as incentive spirometry or intermittent positive pressure breathing (IPPB).
   4. **Emotional state**
      a. Ask patient to describe feelings.
      b. Note patient's physical response during questions.

IV. REVIEWING THE PATIENT CHART

A. After patient has been admitted and a need for respiratory care determined, the chart should be reviewed for the following:
   1. Patient history
   2. Physical exam on admission
   3. Current vital signs
      a. Heart rate
      b. Respiratory rate — if rate remains elevated or there is little or no change in the patient's respiratory distress, the respiratory care practitioner should recommend modifications in the prescribed oxygen therapy — for example, increase in fractional concentration of inspired oxygen (FIO_2), placement on continuous positive airway pressure (CPAP), or institution of mechanical ventilation (see Chapter 9, "Ventilator Management").
      c. Blood pressure — decrease in blood pressure may indicate excessive positive end-expiratory pressure (PEEP) levels requiring a decrease in the prescribed level of PEEP (see Chapter 9, "Ventilator Management").
   4. Current respiratory care orders
      a. Oxygen delivery device
      b. Percentage or liter flow of oxygen
      c. Type of ventilator and prescribed parameters
      d. Frequency and duration of prescribed treatments
      e. Medications ordered with treatment
   5. Patient progress notes
   6. Laboratory values
      a. **Red blood cell (RBC) count** — normal value is 4 million to 6 million/mm³ of blood. A decreased RBC count indicates deficient oxygen-carrying capacity, and the patient should be given blood.
      b. **White blood cell (WBC) count** — normal value is 5,000 to 10,000/mm³ of blood. An increased WBC indicates infection. The respiratory care practitioner may recommend a chest x-ray or sputum culture to determine lung involvement.
      c. **Arterial blood gas values** — abnormal values

in arterial oxygenation (Pa_{O_2}) and/or alveolar ventilation (Pa_{CO_2}) indicate changes in oxygen therapy or ventilatory parameters (see Chapter 8, "Arterial Blood Gas Interpretation," and Chapter 9, "Ventilator Management").

7. Pulmonary function results
   a. Determine severity of lung dysfunction
   b. Determine obstructive or restrictive abnormalities
   c. Recommendation of pre- and postbronchodilator studies to determine responsiveness

REFERENCES

Eubanks D, Bone R. *Comprehensive Respiratory Care.* 2nd ed. St. Louis: CV Mosby; 1990.

Farzan S. *A Concise Handbook of Respiratory Diseases.* 2nd ed. Reston, VA: Prentice-Hall Publishing; 1985.

Scanlan C, Spearman C. *Egan's Fundamentals of Respiratory Care.* 5th ed. St. Louis: CV Mosby; 1990.

PRETEST ANSWERS

1. B
2. A
3. C
4. B
5. D
6. B

Oxygen and Medical Gas Therapy

PRETEST QUESTIONS*

1. After a regulator is attached to an E cylinder and is turned on, a whistling noise is heard from the cylinder. What may be the cause of this?

A. The plastic cover on the cylinder gauge is missing.
B. The regulator is attached too tightly.
C. The plastic washer is missing.
D. The regulator is not compensated for pressure.

2. How long will an E cylinder with 1000 psig last running at 5 L/min until it reaches 200 psig?

A. 21 minutes
B. 45 minutes
C. 56 minutes
D. 1 hour and 10 minutes

3. All of the following statements concerning a Bourdon gauge are true EXCEPT

A. It is not compensated for pressure.
B. Its flow reading is not affected when placed in a horizontal position.
C. It measures pressure directly and flow indirectly.
D. The gauge reads lower than the amount the patient actually receives.

4. The physician orders 28% oxygen to be administered to a COPD patient. Which device will most accurately achieve this?

A. nasal cannula
B. simple oxygen mask
C. Venturi mask
D. nonrebreathing mask

5. A patient is set up on 40% flow-by, and during inspiration mist is not visible exiting the T-tube reservoir. What should the respiratory care practitioner recommend?

A. Increase the nebulizer flow.
B. Add water to the nebulizer.
C. Shorten the T-tube reservoir.
D. Decrease the nebulizer flow.

6. After turning a flowmeter completely off, you notice there is still some bubbling present in the humidifier. This is most likely caused by which of the following?

A. The flowmeter is uncompensated.
B. The flowmeter housing is cracked.
C. Water has entered the flowmeter.
D. The flowmeter has a faulty valve seat.

___
*See answers at the end of the chapter.

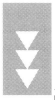

Oxygen and Medical Gas Therapy

I. STORAGE AND CONTROL OF MEDICAL GASES

A. Storage of medical gases and cylinder characteristics
   1. Cylinders are constructed of **chrome molybdenum steel.**
   2. Gas cylinders are stored at high pressures, with a **full oxygen cylinder containing 2200 psig pressure.**
   3. Cylinders are produced in various sizes; the most common sizes used for oxygen storage are the "H" cylinder and the "E" cylinder.
      a. The **H cylinder holds 244 cubic feet (6900 liters) of oxygen.**
      b. The **E cylinder, used for transport, holds 22 cubic feet (622 liters) of oxygen.**
   4. Cylinder valves allow attachment of regulators to remove the gas from the cylinder at various flowrates.
   5. Valves are constructed to allow connection of only one type of gas regulator (e.g., an oxygen regulator will not attach to a helium cylinder). Improper connection is also prevented by the use of cylinder/regulator safety systems.
      a. **Large cylinders use the American Standard Safety System (ASSS).**
      b. **Small cylinders use the Pin Index Safety System (PISS).**
   6. Safety relief devices on cylinder valves allow for the escape of excess gas should the pressure in the cylinder increase. There are two types of safety relief devices.
      a. Frangible disk — breaks at 3000 psig
      b. Fusible plug — melts at 170°F
   7. The Compressed Gas Association (CGA) developed a color-code system for cylinders to distinguish the various gases.

Gas	*Color of Cylinder*
Oxygen	Green
	White (internationally)
Helium	Brown
Carbon dioxide	Gray
Nitrous oxide	Light blue
Cyclopropane	Orange
Ethylene	Red
Air	Yellow
Carbon dioxide/oxygen	Gray and green
Helium/oxygen	Brown and green

8. Cylinder markings

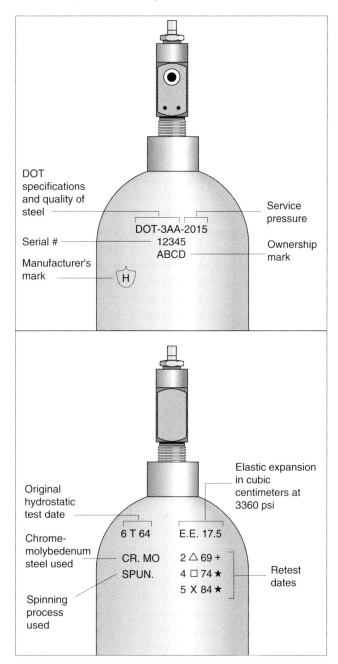

DOT specifications and quality of steel

Serial #

Manufacturer's mark

DOT-3AA-2015
12345
ABCD

H

Service pressure

Ownership mark

Original hydrostatic test date

Chrome-molybedenum steel used

Spinning process used

6 T 64

CR. MO

SPUN.

E.E. 17.5

2 △ 69 +

4 □ 74 ★

5 X 84 ★

Elastic expansion in cubic centimeters at 3360 psi

Retest dates

9. Cylinder testing
   a. Cylinders are visually tested by suspending a light bulb inside and looking for corrosion.
   b. Cylinders are **hydrostatically tested every 5 or 10 years** depending on the cylinder marking. **A star next to the latest test date denotes a 10-year period before the next test must be done.**
   c. Hydrostatic testing determines:
      (1) Wall stress
      (2) Cylinder expansion
      (3) Leaks

10. Bulk oxygen storage
    a. Liquid oxygen is stored in large thermos-type tanks at approximately 250 psig.
    b. Liquid bulk systems consist of cylindrical or spherical-shaped containers with capacities of up to 151 cubic feet liquid oxygen. This converts to 130,000 cubic feet of gaseous oxygen (equal to 533 H cylinders!)

NOTE: As liquid oxygen changes from its liquid state to gas, it expands 860 times. In other words, 1 cubic foot of liquid oxygen when warmed above its boiling point (-297°F), converts to 860 cubic feet gaseous oxygen.

    c. The process by which liquid O_2 is converted to gas in a bulk system or portable system is by the use of **vaporizers**. The vaporizers extract liquid O_2 from the reservoir and heat it, converting it to a gas.
    d. Oxygen may be stored in gaseous bulk systems. There are three types of gas bulk systems:
       (1) Standard cylinder type (manifold system)
           (a) Tanks (H cylinders) are connected together by a manifold, which essentially converts the individual tanks into one continuous supply.
           (b) The manifold mechanism contains pressure-reducing valves, flow controls, and alarms that warn if the supply is getting low.
           (c) Most commonly, six or more tanks are manifolded together and, as they empty, are simply replaced with full tanks.
       (2) Fixed cylinder type
           (a) Large banks of H cylinders, sometimes as many as 75 tanks, are permanently fixed at a station.
           (b) When half of the tanks become empty, they are refilled at their location by a truck that contains liquid O_2.
       (3) Trailer units
           (a) Tanks of various sizes are mounted on trailers and are towed to an area near the hospital and connected to a circuit which runs to the hospital.
           (b) Up to 30 cylinders may be utilized, and when they are empty, the trailer is replaced with full cylinders.

B. Control of medical gases
1. Regulators are devices attached to the cylinder valve to:
   a. Regulate flow
   b. Reduce cylinder pressure to working pressure (50 psig)
2. The reducing valve may be:
   a. Single stage — one pressure relief device
   b. Double stage — two pressure relief devices
   c. Triple stage — three pressure relief devices
3. Regulators may be preset or adjustable.
4. Operation of a **preset regulator**

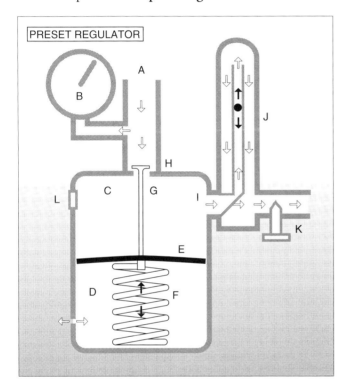

PRESET REGULATOR

a. High-pressure gas enters the inlet (A) of the reducing valve past an inlet valve (H) into the pressure chamber (C). The valve stem (G) is also shown. Cylinder gauge (B) indicates cylinder pressure in psig.
b. Gas pushes down on the diaphragm (E). As the gas pressure overcomes the pressure on the spring (F) attached to the diaphragm, it moves downward, pulling with it the valve that closes off gas flow into the pressure chamber. The spring is located in the ambient chamber (D).
c. As gas exits the pressure chamber through the outlet (I), pressure again drops in the chamber, and the spring, diaphragm, and valve move upward to allow gas to enter the chamber again.
d. In essence, the spring and diaphragm are

continually moving up and down as gas leaves the chamber and goes through the flowmeter (J) and needle valve (K).
e. Excessive pressure in the pressure chamber is vented through a pressure relief valve (L).
f. The spring tension on this type of regulator is **preset at 50 psig.**
5. Operation of an **adjustable regulator**

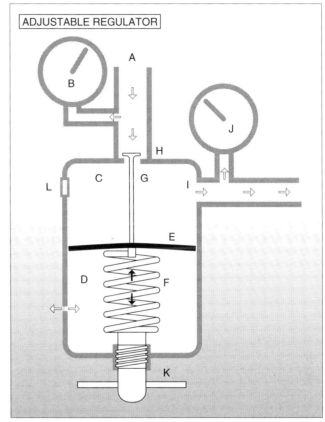

ADJUSTABLE REGULATOR

a. This is an example of a Bourdon gauge regulator.
b. Works the same as the preset regulator except the spring tension is adjustable by the user
6. Technical problems associated with reducing valves and regulators
   a. Dust or debris from the cylinder valve entering the regulator may rupture the diaphragm. **Always "crack" the cylinder prior to attaching a regulator by turning the cylinder valve on and off quickly.**
   b. Constant pressure from gas trapped in the pressure chamber after the cylinder is turned off may rupture the diaphragm. Always vent out gas in the regulator by opening the needle valve after the cylinder is turned off.
   c. A hole in the diaphragm will result in a continuous leak into the ambient chamber

and out the vent hole, causing failure of the regulator.

   d. A weak spring could result in diaphragm vibration, causing inadequate flows due to premature closing of the inlet valve.

   e. When attaching a regulator to a small cylinder, make sure the plastic washer is in place or gas will be heard leaking around the cylinder valve outlet and regulator inlet.

  7. **Calculating how long cylinder contents will last**

$$\text{Minutes remaining in cylinder} = \frac{\text{cylinder pressure} \times \text{cylinder factor}}{\text{flowrate}}$$

Cylinder factors: $\quad$ H cylinder = 3.14 L/psig
$\qquad\qquad\qquad$ E cylinder = 0.28 L/psig

EXAMPLE: Calculate how long a full H cylinder will last running at 8 L/min.

$$\frac{2200 \text{ psig} \times 3.14 \text{ L/psig}}{8 \text{ L/min}} = \frac{6908}{8} = \frac{863.5 \text{ min}}{60} = \textbf{14.39 hr}$$

EXAMPLE: An E cylinder of oxygen contains 1800 psig. If the respiratory care practitioner runs the cylinder at 4 L/min through a nasal cannula, how long will the contents last until the cylinder reaches 200 psig?

$$\frac{(1800 \text{ psig} - 200 \text{ psig}) \times 0.28 \text{ L/psig}}{4 \text{ L/min}} = \frac{448}{4} = \textbf{112 min}$$

$$\frac{112 \text{ min}}{60} = \textbf{1.9 hr}$$

  8. **Flowmeters**
   a. **Uncompensated flowmeter**

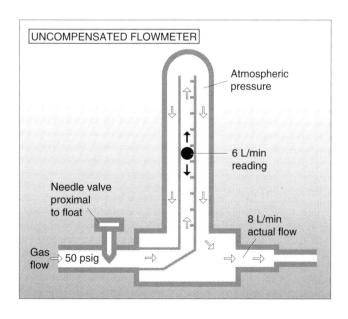

    (1) Needle valve is located proximal to (before) the float; therefore, atmospheric pressure is in the tube. Any back pressure in the tube affects the rise of the float.

    (2) When a restriction (e.g., a humidifier or nebulizer) is attached to the outlet, back pressure results in an inaccurate reading. The flowmeter reads lower than the amount the patient actually receives.

    (3) Should not be used clinically

   b. **Compensated flowmeter**

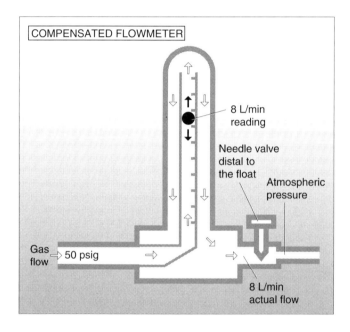

    (1) The needle valve is located distal to (after) the float; therefore, 50 psig is in the tube, and only back pressure exceeding that will affect the rise of the float.

    (2) The flowmeter reads accurately with an attachment such as a humidifier or nebulizer on the outlet.

    (3) There are three ways to determine if a flowmeter is compensated for pressure.
      (a) Labeled as such on the flowmeter
      (b) Needle valve is located after the float.
      (c) Float jumps when the flowmeter is plugged into wall outlet while turned off.

    (4) Flowmeter outlets utilize the **Diameter Index Safety System (DISS)**, as do all gas administration units that operate at **less than 200 psig**, to avoid attachment to the wrong gas source.

(5) If the flowmeter is turned completely off, but gas is still bubbling through the humidifier or gas is still heard coming out the flowmeter, this indicates a faulty valve seat and the flowmeter should be replaced.

c. **Bourdon gauge**

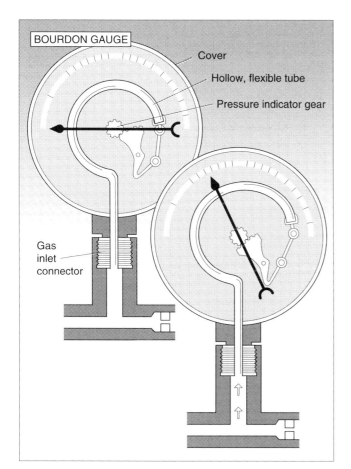

BOURDON GAUGE

Cover

Hollow, flexible tube

Pressure indicator gear

Gas inlet connector

(1) The Bourdon gauge is actually a pressure gauge that has been calibrated in liters per minute. **It is not compensated for back pressure.**

(2) When a humidifier or nebulizer is attached to its outlet, back pressure is generated into the gauge (which measures pressure) and **reads higher than the amount the patient is actually receiving.**

(3) The gauge's working mechanism operates by gas entering the hollow, flexible, question-mark-shaped tube. The tube tends to straighten as pressure is applied to it. A gear mechanism is attached to the tube, and as the tube

straightens it rotates a needle indicator denoting the pressure (flow).

(4) The advantage of the Bourdon gauge is that it is not position dependent like Thorpe tube flowmeters.

9. **Air compressors**

a. Used to provide medical air through either portable air compressors or large medical air piping systems.

b. Three types of air compressors are generally used.

(1) Piston type

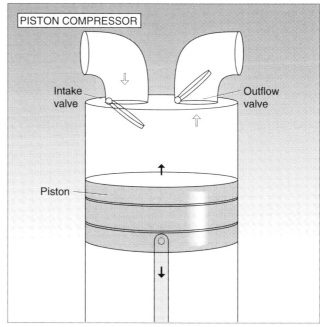

PISTON COMPRESSOR

Intake valve

Outflow valve

Piston

(a) As piston drops, gas is drawn in through a one-way intake valve. On the upstroke, the intake valve closes and gas exits through a one-way outflow valve.

(b) Air is drawn into the compressor and travels to a reservoir tank. From this tank the air passes through a drier to remove the moisture and a pressure-reducing valve that reduces the pressure to 50 psi to power the compressed-air wall outlet.

(c) Seen most commonly on large medical air piping systems.

(2) Diaphragm type

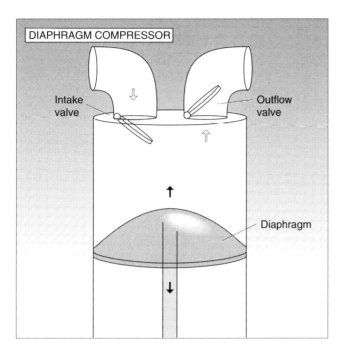

DIAPHRAGM COMPRESSOR

Intake valve

Outflow valve

Diaphragm

(a) A diaphragm is used instead of a piston.
(b) On the downstroke, the flexible diaphragm bends downward, drawing air in through a one-way intake valve. Air is forced out the one-way outflow valve on the upstroke.
(c) Used commonly on oxygen concentrators.

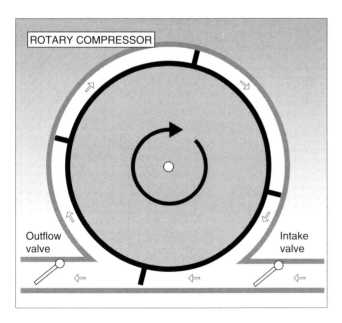

ROTARY COMPRESSOR

Outflow valve

Intake valve

(3) Rotary type
(a) The rotor acts like a fan, pushing air from one area to another. As the rotor turns, gas is drawn into one side and forced out the other.
(b) Used in the MA-1 ventilator.

II. OXYGEN THERAPY

A. Indications for oxygen therapy
1. Treat hypoxemia
2. Decrease the work of breathing
3. Reduce myocardial work
B. **Signs and symptoms of hypoxemia**
1. Tachycardia
2. Dyspnea
3. Cyanosis
4. Impairment of special senses
5. Headache
6. Mental disturbance
7. Slight hyperventilation

NOTE: It is important to remember that hypoxemia may worsen and ventilation/perfusion (V/Q) mismatching will increase if patients with lung conditions are not properly positioned. Since blood flow is affected by gravity, positioning the patient with the diseased area of the lung down (dependent position) will cause an increased perfusion to the diseased lung, causing decreased Pa_{O_2} levels and an increased V/Q mismatch. Therefore, position the patient's bad lung area up (independent position) to decrease perfusion to that area in order to increase Pa_{O_2} and decrease V/Q mismatching.

C. Complications of oxygen therapy
1. Respiratory depression — most affected is the COPD patient breathing on "hypoxic drive" mechanism. **Maintain Pa_{O_2} at 50 to 60 mm Hg.**
2. Atelectasis — high oxygen concentrations in the lung wash out nitrogen in the lung and reduce the production of surfactant, leading to atelectasis. Maintain F_{IO_2} below 0.5 to 0.6.
3. Oxygen toxicity — high oxygen concentrations result in toxicity to lung tissue due to increased oxygen free radicals. This leads to acute respiratory distress syndrome (ARDS). Maintain F_{IO_2} below 0.5 to 0.6.

4. Retrolental fibroplasia (neonatal retinopathy) — caused by **high Pa_{O_2} levels** in infants, leading to blindness. More common in premature infants. **Maintain Pa_{O_2} below 100 mm Hg.** Normal Pa_{O_2} in infants is 50 to 70 mm Hg.
5. Reduced mucociliary activity — maintain F_{IO_2} below 0.5 to 0.6.

D. Normal Pa_{O_2} values by age

Age (years)	*Normal* Pa_{O_2}
<60	80 mm Hg
70	70 mm Hg
80	60 mm Hg
90	50 mm Hg

E. Four types of hypoxia
 1. **Hypoxemic hypoxia**
  a. Caused by lack of oxygen in the blood due to:
   (1) Inadequate oxygen in the inspired air — giving oxygen beneficial
   (2) Alveolar hypoventilation — oxygen alone may not be beneficial
   (3) Atelectasis — oxygen alone not beneficial
   (4) Pulmonary edema — high oxygen percentage may be beneficial
   (5) Ventilation/perfusion mismatch — oxygen may be beneficial
   (6) Anatomic right-to-left shunt — oxygen not beneficial
  b. **If a normal Pa_{O_2} cannot be maintained with a 60% oxygen mask,** a large shunt is probable and should not be treated with higher oxygen concentrations. **CPAP should be administered (if the Pa_{CO_2} is normal or low).**
 2. **Anemic hypoxia**
  a. Capacity of blood to carry oxygen is decreased due to:
   (1) Decreased hemoglobin level — give RBCs
   (2) Carbon monoxide poisoning — use 100% oxygen
   (3) Excessive blood loss — give blood
   (4) Methemoglobin — results from toxic drug reaction

   (5) Iron deficiency — increase iron intake, give blood
  b. Carbon monoxide poisoning must be treated with 100% oxygen or hyperbaric oxygen if available. The higher the Pa_{O_2}, the more readily hemoglobin will release the bound carbon monoxide. This allows for more available hemoglobin for oxygen to bind with.
  c. Carbon monoxide's affinity for hemoglobin is 200 to 250 times greater than that of oxygen.
  d. Normal hemoglobin (Hb) level is 12 to 16 gm/100 ml of blood.
  e. Oxygen is carried in the blood two ways:
   (1) Bound to hemoglobin (1.34 x Hb x SaO_2)
   (2) Dissolved in plasma (0.003 x Pa_{O_2})

NOTE: The sum of these two equals the total oxygen content in milliliters and is the most effective method to determine a patient's oxygen-carrying capacity.

 3. **Stagnant (circulatory) hypoxia**
  a. The oxygen content and carrying capacity are normal, but capillary perfusion is diminished as a result of:
   (1) Decreased heart rate
   (2) Decreased cardiac output
   (3) Shock
   (4) Emboli
  b. May be seen as a localized problem (peripheral cyanosis due to exposure to cold weather)
 4. **Histotoxic hypoxia**
  a. The oxidative enzyme mechanism of the cell is impaired as a result of:
   (1) Cyanide poisoning
   (2) Alcohol poisoning
  b. Rarely accompanied by hypoxemia but by increased venous P_{O_2} levels
F. **Oxygen delivery devices**
 1. **Low-flow oxygen systems** — an oxygen delivery device that does not meet the patient's inspiratory flow demands; therefore, room air is entrained by the patient to make up the difference. Normal spontaneous inspiratory flowrate is 25 to 30 L/min. Therefore, any device delivering less than 25 L/min will require the patient to entrain room air into the device. The following devices are connected to **humidifiers**. (In some areas, humidifiers are not used if less than 5 L/min is delivered.)

a. **Nasal catheter**

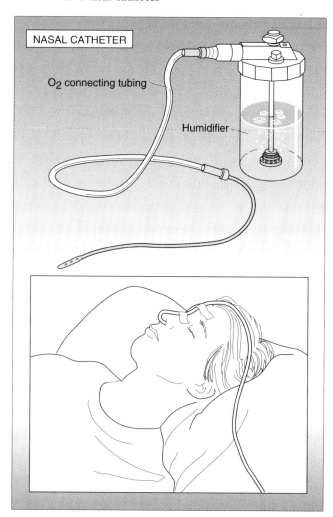

b. **Nasal cannula**

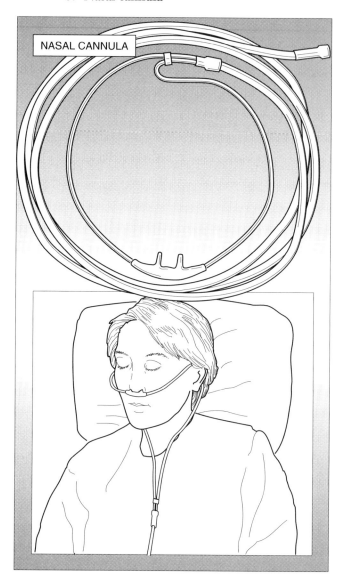

(1) Delivers oxygen percentages of 24% to 44% at flows of 1 to 6 L/min (about 4% increase per liter)

(2) Catheter should be lubricated with water-soluble gel and inserted nasally to just above the uvula. Catheter may be measured from patient's nose to ear to establish correct placement if direct visualization is not possible.

(3) If catheter inserted too far, air swallowing and gastric distention may result.

(4) Change catheter to alternate nostril every 8 hours.

(1) Delivers oxygen percentages of 24% to 44% at flows of 1 to 6 L/min (about 4% increase per liter)

(2) Much better tolerated by the patient than a nasal catheter

(3) Nasal catheters and cannulas are available in infant sizes and are most commonly used for long-term oxygen therapy in the treatment of bronchopulmonary dysplasia (BPD) and other chronic diseases.

(4) The flowmeters used to deliver oxygen through the catheter or cannula to infants or pediatric patients should be calibrated into small increments so that one-fourth or one-half liter per minute is available.

c. **Simple oxygen mask**

d. **Partial rebreathing mask**

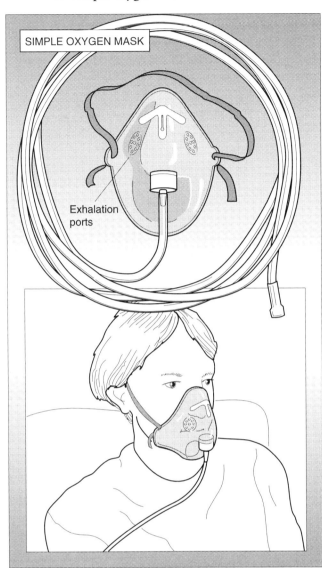

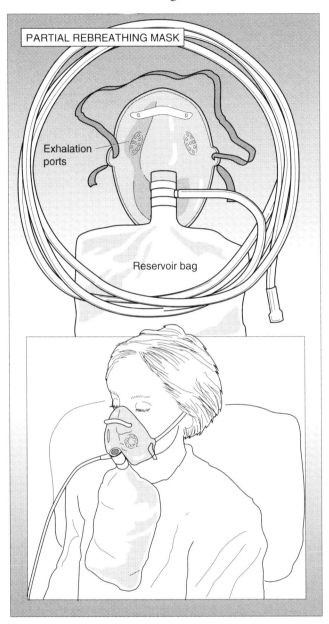

(1) Delivers oxygen percentages of 35% to 55% at flows of 6 to 10 L/min
(2) Minimum flowrate of 6 L/min is needed to prevent buildup of exhaled carbon dioxide in the mask.

(1) Delivers oxygen percentages of 35% to 60% at flows of 8 to 15 L/min
(2) Flowrate must be sufficient to keep the reservoir bag at least one-third to half full at all times.
(3) Ensure that the patient is not positioned so that a kink could develop in the reservoir bag. Lower oxygen percentage would result.

e. Nonrebreathing mask

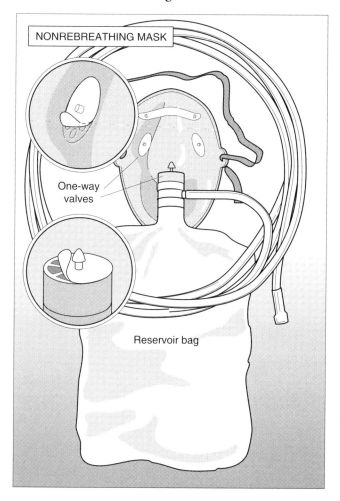

NONREBREATHING MASK

One-way valves

Reservoir bag

(1) Delivers oxygen percentages of 75% to 100% at flows of 8 to 15 L/min
(2) Flowrate must be sufficient to keep the reservoir bag at least one-third to half full at all times.
(3) The nonrebreather is equipped with a one-way flutter valve between the mask and the reservoir bag that does not allow exhaled gases into the reservoir bag.
(4) One-way flutter valves are located on side ports of the mask to prevent room air entrainment. If one valve is used, FIO_2 decreases and the mask is considered low flow; if both valves are used, FIO_2 increases and it is considered a high-flow device.
(5) Ensure that the reservoir bag does not become kinked, especially if both exhalation ports have one-way valves, as no room air would be available to the patient. (For this reason, one valve is often left off.)

NOTE: **If the reservoir bag does not deflate during the patient's inspiration, the one-way valve between the bag and mask may be sticking or the mask may not be fitting tight enough. If the bag totally deflates during inspiration, the flowrate is too low and must be increased to keep the bag one-half to one-third full.**

f. Low-flow oxygen devices are adequate for use only if the patient meets the following criteria:
  (1) Tidal volume of 300 to 700 ml
  (2) Respiratory rate less than 25/min
  (3) Regular and consistent ventilatory pattern
g. **Any patient requiring supplemental oxygen who does not meet these criteria should be placed on a high-flow oxygen delivery device (see below).**
h. The percentage of oxygen delivered by a low-flow device is variable depending upon the patient's tidal volume, respiratory rate, inspiratory time, and ventilatory pattern.
2. **High-flow devices** — devices that provide all the total inspiratory flow required by the patient. They provide relatively accurate and consistent oxygen percentages. With the exception of the Venturi mask, these devices are attached to **nebulizers.**

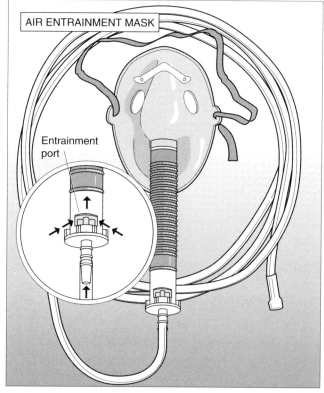

AIR ENTRAINMENT MASK

Entrainment port

a. **Venturi mask (air entrainment mask) — 24% to 50%**
   (1) Increasing the flowrate on the device will not alter the F_{IO_2}; the jet size and entrainment port alter the F_{IO_2}.
      (a) Larger entrainment port — more air entrained — lower F_{IO_2}
      (b) Smaller entrainment port — less air entrained — higher F_{IO_2}
      (c) Larger jet size — less air entrained — higher F_{IO_2}
      (d) Smaller jet size — more air entrained — lower F_{IO_2}

NOTE: It is important to prevent the entrainment port from becoming occluded (by patient's hand, bedsheet, etc.), as this will decrease the amount of air entrainment and thus increase the delivered oxygen percentage.

   (2) Air:oxygen entrainment ratios

Air:Oxygen Ratio	Oxygen Percentage
25:1	24%
10:1	28%
8:1	30%
5:1	35%
3:1	40%
1.7:1	50%
1:1	60%

These ratios may be calculated by the following formula:

$$\frac{100 - x}{x - 20^*} = \frac{\text{parts air entrained}}{\text{one part oxygen}}$$

EXAMPLE: Calculate the air:oxygen ratio for 40%.

$$\frac{100 - 40}{40 - 20} = \frac{60}{20} = \frac{3}{1} \text{ or 3:1 ratio}$$

This means that for every liter of oxygen (source gas) delivered from the flowmeter, 3 liters of air are entrained into the device.

   (3) **Calculating total flow**
If a Venturi mask is set on 40% and a flowrate of 8 L/min, the total flow delivered would be:

*Use 21 with percentages less than 40%.

8 L/min of oxygen
24 L/min of air (8 × 3)
32 L/min total flow

FASTER METHOD: Add the ratio parts and multiply by the flow.
ratio parts 3 + 1 = 4
4 × 8 = 32 L/min

EXAMPLE: A Venturi mask is set on 24% and a flow of 4 L/min. Calculate the total flow.

$$\frac{100 - 24}{24 - 21} = \frac{76}{3} = \frac{25}{1} = \textbf{25:1 air:oxygen ratio}$$

4 L/min of oxygen
100 L/min of air (25 × 4)
104 L/min total flow
sum of ratio parts × flow

(25 + 1) = 26 × 4 = **104 L/min**

b. **Aerosol mask**

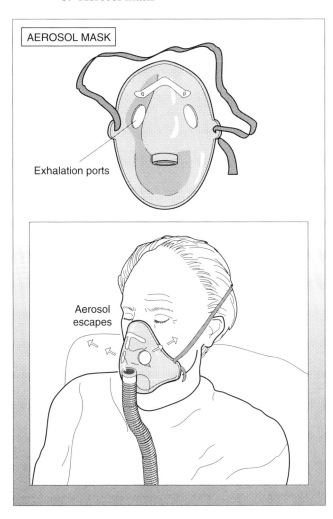

AEROSOL MASK

Exhalation ports

Aerosol escapes

     (1) Delivers oxygen percentages of 21% to 60% (depending on nebulizer setting) at flows of 8 to 15 L/min (on flowmeter)

     (2) If the nebulizer is set on 100%, the device would not likely meet the patient's inspiratory flow demands. Room air would be entrained, decreasing F_{IO_2}.

     (3) <u>Mist should be visible at all times flowing out the exhalation ports to ensure adequate flows.</u>

  c. **Face tent**

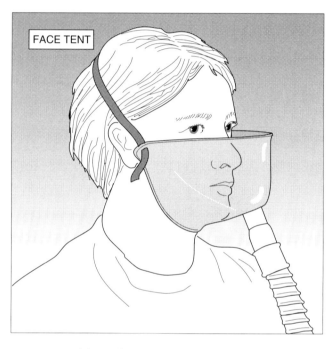

FACE TENT

     (1) Delivers oxygen percentages of 21% to 40% (depending on nebulizer setting) at flows of 8 to 15 L/min

     (2) Used primarily on patients with facial trauma and burns or those who cannot tolerate a mask

  d. **T-tube flow-by or Briggs adaptor**

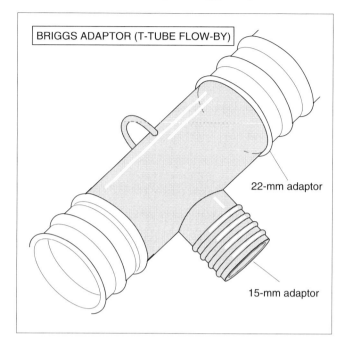

BRIGGS ADAPTOR (T-TUBE FLOW-BY)

22-mm adaptor

15-mm adaptor

     (1) Delivers oxygen percentages of 21% to 100% (depending on nebulizer setting) at flows of 8 to 15 L/min

     (2) Used on the intubated or tracheostomy patient

     (3) A 50-cc piece of reservoir tubing should be attached to the opposite end of the T-piece. This prevents air entrainment during inspiration.

     (4) <u>Adequate flows are ensured by visible mist flowing out of the 50-cc reservoir at all times.</u>

e. **Tracheostomy mask (collar)**

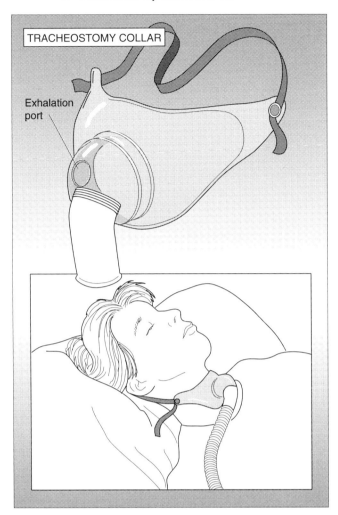

f. **Oxygen hood**

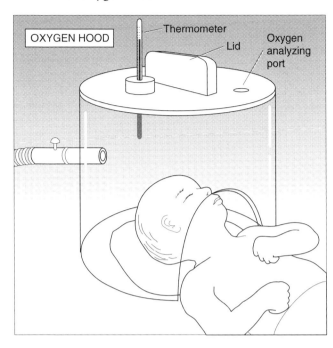

(1) Delivers oxygen percentages of 35% to 60% (depending on nebulizer setting) at flows of 10 to 15 L/min

(2) Adequate flows are ensured by visible mist flowing out of the exhalation port at all times.

(3) Mask should fit directly over the tracheostomy tube.

(1) A small, clear plastic enclosure placed over an infant's head to deliver oxygen and aerosol

(2) It is best to heat the delivered gas, as cool gas can cause an increase in the infant's oxygen consumption.

(3) Some hoods have been designed so that oxygen concentrations have a "layering" effect. The highest concentration is near the bottom of the hood.

(4) Care must be taken to closely monitor and control the delivered oxygen percentage, aerosol temperature, and body water of the infant.

(5) The temperature of the inside of the hood and the oxygen concentration should be monitored continuously through separate ports in the top of the hood. (The oxygen concentration to be analyzed should be as close to the infant as possible.)

(6) Large-bore aerosol tubing from a nebulizer attaches to the back of the hood to deliver oxygen/aerosol. High noise level from the incoming gas is a hazard with this device.

g. **Oxygen tent**

(1) Delivers oxygen percentages of 21% to 50% at flows of 15 L/min or higher

(2) Used primarily on children with croup or pneumonia

(3) Not an ideal oxygen delivery device owing to high incidence of leaks and reduced oxygen percentage when the tent is opened for patient care

(4) A fire hazard exists if electrical devices or toys that may spark with friction are left in the tent.

G. **Important points concerning high-flow devices**

1. A high-flow device set on 60% or higher may deliver a total flow of less than 25 to 30 L/min, which may not meet the patient's inspiratory flow demands. It essentially acts as a low-flow device, with the patient breathing in room air to make up the difference. This means the oxygen setting on the device is no longer accurate and the patient is receiving less delivered oxygen.

2. To ensure adequate flows on a device set on 60% or higher, use two flowmeters connected together in-line.

3. To ensure adequate flows, set the flowmeter to a rate that will deliver a total flow of at **least 40 L/min.**

4. A restriction, such as kinked aerosol tubing or water in the tubing, causes a back pressure into the nebulizer, decreasing the amount of air entrainment and thus increasing the oxygen percentage.

5. Increasing the flowrate on a high-flow device will not increase the delivered F_{IO_2}; it will only increase the total flow.

H. **Calculating F_{IO_2}**

$$F_{IO_2} = \frac{\text{oxygen flow} + (\text{air flow} \times 0.2)}{\text{total flow}}$$

EXAMPLE: A nebulizer set on the 40% dilution mode and connected to an oxygen flowmeter running at 10 L/min has an air bleed-in of 6 L/min downstream. Calculate the F_{IO_2}.

oxygen flow	=	10 L/min
air flow	=	30 L/min (entrained through nebulizer)
air flow	=	6 L/min (bleed-in)
total flow	=	46 L/min

$$F_{IO_2} = \frac{10 + (36 \times 0.2)}{46} = \frac{10 + 7.2}{46} = \frac{17.2}{46} = 0.37$$

I. **Oxygen blenders**

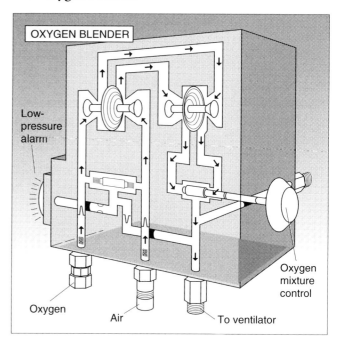

1. These devices utilize 50-psi gas sources to mix or blend oxygen and compressed air proportionately to deliver oxygen percentages of 21% to 100% at flowrates of 2 to 100 L/min.

2. A blender consists of pressure-regulating valves that regulate oxygen and air inlet pressure, a mixture control (precision metering device), and an audible alarm system that sounds if there is a drop in inlet pressure.

3. Blenders provide a stable F_{IO_2} as long as the outlet flow exceeds the patient's inspiratory flow demands.

III. OXYGEN ANALYZERS

A. **Physical analyzer (paramagnetic)**
1. Utilizes the Pauling principle
2. More closely measures partial pressure of oxygen
3. Reading is affected by higher altitude.
4. Beckman D-2 is an example of a physical analyzer.

B. **Electrical analyzer**
1. Utilizes the "wheatstone bridge" and the principle of thermal conduction
2. More closely measures oxygen percentage
3. Has a slow response time
4. Mira is an example of an electrical analyzer.

C. Electrochemical analyzer
1. **Galvanic cell type (utilizes a fuel cell)**
   a. Electrolyte gel is used to chemically reduce oxygen-to-electron flow.
   b. Uses a Clark electrode and measures partial pressure
   c. Reading is affected by water, positive pressure, high altitude, torn membrane, or lack of electrolyte gel.
   d. Teledyne and Hudson are examples of the galvanic cell electrochemical analyzer.
2. **Polarographic type**
   a. A battery polarizes the electrodes to allow oxygen reduction to occur, giving off electron flow.
   b. Uses the Clark electrode and more accurately measures partial pressures
   c. Reading is affected by water, positive pressure, high altitude, torn membrane, or lack of electrolyte gel.
   d. Electrodes last longer on the galvanic cell but the polarographic type has a quicker response time.
   e. IL and Ohio are examples of the polarographic electrochemical analyzer.

IV. CO-OXIMETRY (CARBON MONOXIDE OXIMETER)

A. This procedure requires an arterial blood sample to be obtained. The blood is analyzed through a blood gas analyzer with spectrophotometric capabilities.
B. This type of oximeter is capable of measuring the amount of hemoglobin (Hb), oxyhemoglobin (amount of O_2 combined with Hb), and carboxyhemoglobin (amount of carbon monoxide combined with Hb).
C. It is the CO-oximeter that is utilized to determine the amount of CO present in the blood in victims of smoke inhalation or exhaust fume inhalation.

NOTE: Pulse oximeters do not accurately reflect the amount of CO in the blood. In fact, they read erroneously high, as they cannot determine what is bound to the Hb—oxygen or carbon monoxide. A victim of a house fire may present in the emergency room with a 98% to 100% oxygen saturation obtained from a pulse oximeter (Sp_{O_2}), when indeed the patient is severely hypoxic. The oximeter calculates that some gas is bound to hemoglobin in a high percentage, but in this case, it is not oxygen.

D. Carboxyhemoglobin is usually expressed as a percentage of total hemoglobin.
E. Carboxyhemoglobin levels as high as 10% may be seen in heavy smokers, but higher levels are measured in victims who have inhaled large amounts of smoke or car fumes.
F. Symptoms of CO poisoning:

Carboxyhemoglobin level concentration (%)	Signs and Symptoms
0-10	None
10-20	Headache, mild dyspnea
20-40	Headache, dyspnea, vomiting, muscle weakness, dizziness, visual impairment
40-60	tachycardia, tachypnea, syncope, coma, seizures, irregular breathing pattern
>60	shock, coma, apnea, death

REFERENCES

Eubanks D, Bone R. *Comprehensive Respiratory Care.* 2nd ed. St. Louis: CV Mosby; 1990.

McPherson SP. *Respiratory Therapy Equipment.* 4th ed. St. Louis: CV Mosby; 1990.

Scanlan C, Spearman C. *Egan's Fundamentals of Respiratory Care.* 5th ed. St. Louis: CV Mosby; 1990.

PRETEST ANSWERS

1. C
2. B
3. D
4. C
5. A
6. D

Humidity and Aerosol Therapy

PRETEST QUESTIONS*

1. You occlude the outlet of a bubble humidifier and no noise is heard coming from it. What could be the cause of this?

   I. The humidifier jar is loose.
  II. The humidifier is cracked.
 III. The diffuser is disconnected from the capillary tube.

  A. I only
  B. II only
  C. I and II only
  D. II and III only

2. Which piece of equipment would be needed to set up a tracheostomy collar on a patient?

  A. heated nebulizer
  B. spinning disk nebulizer
  C. bubble humidifier
  D. pass-over humidifier

3. Which of the following devices will deliver the highest water content?

  A. spinning disk nebulizer
  B. jet nebulizer
  C. bubble humidifier
  D. ultrasonic nebulizer

*See answers at the end of the chapter.

4. While performing oxygen rounds, the respiratory care practitioner notices very little mist coming out of the patient's aerosol mask, which is attached to a heated nebulizer. Which of the following could cause this?

   I. plugged capillary tube
  II. water in the aerosol tubing
 III. low water level in nebulizer
 IV. inadequate flowrate

  A. I and II only
  B. II and III only
  C. II, III, and IV only
  D. I, II, III, and IV

5. The reservoir of a Cascade II humidifier inadvertently runs dry. What will happen when this occurs?

  A. The ventilator to which it is attached will overheat.
  B. The heater will turn off.
  C. The humidifier will melt.
  D. Gas flow through the humidifier will decrease.

6. A patient is set up on a 40% aerosol mask, which when analyzed reads 65%. What is the appropriate action to take?

  A. Increase the nebulizer flow.
  B. Decrease the nebulizer flow.
  C. Drain the water from the aerosol tubing.
  D. Shorten the aerosol tubing.

CHAPTER **3**

Humidity and Aerosol Therapy

I. HUMIDITY THERAPY

A. **Humidity** — water in a gaseous state or vapor. Also called "molecular water" or "invisible moisture."

B. **Clinical uses of humidity**
1. Humidify dry therapeutic gases
2. Provide 100% body humidity of the inspired gas for patients with endotracheal tubes or tracheostomy tubes

NOTE: **The objective of humidity therapy is to compensate for water loss that occurs when dry gas is delivered or when the upper airway is bypassed. Adding "liquid" water or mist to the airway to thin secretions is accomplished by aerosol therapy (discussed later in this chapter).**

C. **Normal airway humidification**
1. Nose — warms, humidifies, and filters inspired air
2. Pharynx, trachea, and bronchial tree — also warm, humidify, and filter inspired air
3. By the time inspired air reaches the oropharynx, it has been warmed to approximately 34°C and is 80% to 90% saturated.
4. By the time the inspired air reaches the carina, it has been warmed to body temperature (37°C) and is 100% saturated.
5. When the inspired air is fully saturated (100%), it holds **44 milligrams of water per liter of gas** and exerts a **water vapor pressure of 47 mm Hg.**

D. **Absolute and relative humidity**
1. **Absolute humidity** — the amount of water in a given volume of gas. Expressed in milligrams per liter.
2. **Relative humidity** — a ratio between the amount of water in a given volume of gas and the amount it is capable of holding at that temperature. **Expressed as a percent. It is measured with the use of a hygrometer.**
3. Relative humidity = $\dfrac{\text{absolute humidity}}{\text{capacity}}$ x 100

EXAMPLE: The amount of moisture in a given volume of gas at 25°C contains 15 mg of water per liter of gas. Calculate the relative humidity. (Note: At 25°C, the air can hold 23.04 mg of water per liter of gas.)

Relative humidity = $\dfrac{15 \text{ mg/L}}{23.04 \text{ mg/L}}$ = 0.65 x 100 = 65%

EXAMPLE: A gas at 27°C has a relative humidity of 45%. Calculate the absolute humidity. (Note: At 27°C, the air can hold 25.75 mg of water per liter of air.)

Absolute humidity = relative humidity x capacity
= 0.45 x 25.75 mg/L = 11.6 mg/L

E. **Body humidity**
1. The relative humidity at body temperature, expressed as a percentage.
2. Body humidity = $\dfrac{\text{absolute humidity}}{44 \text{ mg/L (capacity at body temperature)}}$ x 100

EXAMPLE: If the patient's inspired gas contains 10 mg of water per liter of air, what is the body humidity?

$$\text{Body humidity} = \frac{10 \text{ mg/L}}{44 \text{ mg/L}} = 0.23 \text{ x } 100 = 23\%$$

3. A 23% body humidity indicates that the inspired air is holding only 23% of the water it takes to fully saturate the gas in the airway at body temperature. The body's humidification system will make up the other 77% by the time the air reaches the carina.

F. **Humidity deficit**
1. Inspired air that is not fully saturated at body temperature creates a humidity deficit. This deficit is filled by the body's own humidification system.
2. Humidity deficit may be expressed in milligrams per liter or as a percent.
3. **Humidity deficit = 44 mg/L – absolute humidity**
or when expressed as a percent:

$$\frac{\textbf{Humidity deficit (mg/L)}}{\textbf{44 mg/L}} \textbf{ x 100}$$

EXAMPLE: A patient on T-tube flow-by is inspiring air from an Ohio nebulizer that contains 23 mg of water per liter of air. What is this patient's humidity deficit?

$$\begin{array}{r} 44 \text{ mg/L} \\ - \ 23 \text{ mg/L} \\ \hline 21 \text{ mg/L} \end{array}$$

and as a percent: $\dfrac{21 \text{ mg/L}}{44 \text{ mg/L}} = 0.48 \text{ x } 100 = 48\%$

4. It is important to deliver humidified gas at body temperature to patients with artificial airways that bypass the patient's upper airway.
5. If adequate humidity is not provided, the patient's airway can dry out, leading to thickening of secretions and resulting in increased airway resistance.

6. Delivery of gas that contains **less than 44 mg of water per liter or a water vapor pressure of less than 47 mm Hg to a patient with an E-T tube or tracheostomy tube will tend to dry secretions out, making them thicker and more difficult to mobilize.**

G. **Efficiency of humidifiers** — dependent upon three important factors
1. Time of contact between the gas and water (longer contact time = increased humidity)
2. Surface area involved in gas/water contact (greater surface area involved = increased humidity)
3. Temperature of the gas and water (increased temperature of gas or water = increased humidity)

H. **Types of humidifiers**
1. **Pass-over humidifier** (nonheated humidifier)

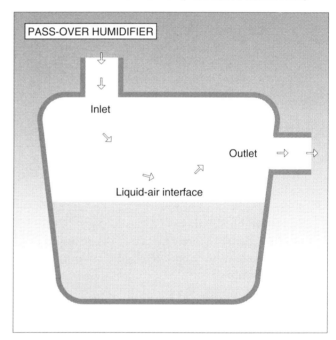

PASS-OVER HUMIDIFIER

Inlet

Outlet

Liquid-air interface

a. Gas simply passes over the surface of the water, picking up moisture and delivering it to the patient.
b. Produces a low-humidity output due to the limited time of gas/water contact and surface area involved
c. Provides a body humidity of approximately 25%

2. **Bubble humidifier** (nonheated humidifier)

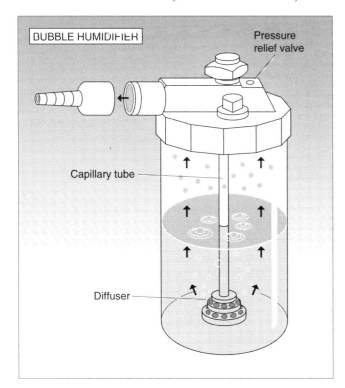

a. The most common type of humidifier used with low-flow oxygen delivery devices
b. Gas flows out of the flowmeter through a tube under the surface of the water and exits through a diffuser at the lower end of the tube.
c. **Provides a body humidity of 35% to 40%**

3. **Wick humidifier** (heated humidifier)

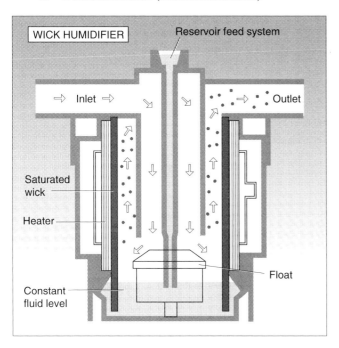

a. Gas from the flowmeter or ventilator enters the humidifier and is exposed to the wick (made of cloth, sponge, or paper) that is partially under the surface of the water.
b. As gas passes the wick, it absorbs water and is delivered to the patient.
c. Because the water bath or the gas is heated, a body humidity approaching 100% is delivered to the patient. It is ideal to use on patients with artificial airways and those on mechanical ventilators.

4. **Cascade humidifier** (heated humidifier)

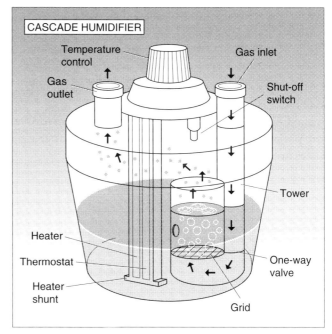

a. Gas travels down the tower and hits the bottom of the jar, which displaces the water upward over a grid, forming a liquid film. The gas travels back up through the grid (from underneath), picking up moisture and delivering it to the patient.
b. Because it is heated, it is capable of delivering the gas at **100% body humidity.**
c. Should the Cascade humidifier be allowed to run dry, the thermostat will automatically turn the heater off, preventing the reservoir from being damaged or hot, dry gas from being delivered to the patient.

I. **Important points concerning humidifiers**
1. Most nonheated humidifiers have a pressure pop-off valve set at **2 psi** (pounds per square inch). After the device is set up, the tubing of the oxygen delivery device (cannula, mask, etc.) should be kinked to obstruct flow. If the pop-off

sounds, there are no leaks. If no sound is heard, all connections should be tightened, as well as the humidifier top.

2. Water levels of all humidifiers should be maintained at the levels marked on the humidifier jar to ensure maximum humidity output.

3. Condensation will occur in the tubing of heated humidifiers. This water should be discarded in a trash container or basin and **never** returned into the humidifier.

4. Inspired gas temperatures should be monitored continuously with an in-line thermometer when using heated humidifiers. The thermometer should be as close to the patient wye as possible.

5. Warm, moist areas such as those within heated humidifiers are breeding grounds for microorganisms (especially *Pseudomonas*). The humidifier should be changed **every 24 hours.**

NOTE: Heated humidifiers are not as likely as heated nebulizers to deliver contaminated moisture to the patient because the small molecular water particles are not able to carry organisms.

J. **Heat moisture exchanger** (HME) (artificial nose)

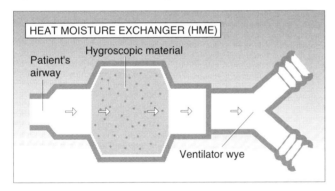

1. This device is placed in-line between the patient and the patient wye of the ventilator circuit.

2. As the patient exhales, gas at body humidity and body temperature enters the HME, heating the hygroscopic filter (made of felt, plastic foam, or cellulose sponge) and condensing water into it. During the next inspiration, gas passes through the HME and is warmed and humidified.

3. Under ideal conditions, the HME can produce 70% to 90% body humidity.

NOTE: If the patient's secretions begin to thicken while using a heat moisture exchanger, a conventional humidifier should be substituted.

4. Over time, the HME may cause a resistance to gas flow because of buildup of water or secretions, observed by increasing peak inspiratory pressures on the ventilator. If all pathologic

reasons are ruled out as the cause of the increased pressures, **the HME should be replaced with a new one.**

II. AEROSOL THERAPY

A. **Aerosol** is defined as water in particulate form or a mist. Nebulizers produce aerosols.

B. **Clinical uses of aerosol therapy**
   1. Improve the mobilization of pulmonary secretions
   2. Administer medications (via hand-held nebulizer or ultrasonic nebulizer)
   3. Prevent dehydration
   4. Following extubation, to prevent or relieve bronchospasm or inflammatory reaction
   5. Hydrate the airways of a tracheostomy patient
   6. Induce cough for sputum collection

C. **Hazards of aerosol therapy**
   1. Bronchospasm — a bronchodilator may decrease the potential of bronchospasm.
   2. Overhydration
   3. Overheating of inspired gas
   4. Tube condensation draining into the airway
   5. Delivery of contaminated aerosol to the patient

D. **Characteristics of aerosol particles**
   1. The ideal particle size for therapeutic use in respiratory care is 0.5 to 3 microns.
   2. Numerous factors affect the penetration and deposition of aerosol particles.
      a. **Gravitational sedimentation** — gravity will have a greater effect on the larger particle, and it will deposit sooner.
      b. **Brownian movement** — affects particles 0.1 micron in size or smaller. Particles in this size range will deposit too soon (possibly in aerosol tubing).
      c. **Inertial impaction** — larger particles have a greater inertia that keeps them moving in a straight direction. They cannot make directional changes in the airway and therefore deposit sooner.
      d. **Hygroscopic properties** — aerosol particles are hygroscopic (retain moisture). As they travel down the airway, they may increase in size as they retain moisture, altering the time in which they deposit.
      e. **Ventilatory pattern** — in order to obtain optimal particle penetration, the patient should be instructed to take **slow, moderately deep breaths, holding each breath for 2 to 3 seconds at the end of inspiration.**

E. **Types of nebulizers (pneumatic)**
1. **Mechanical nebulizer** (entrainment nebulizer)

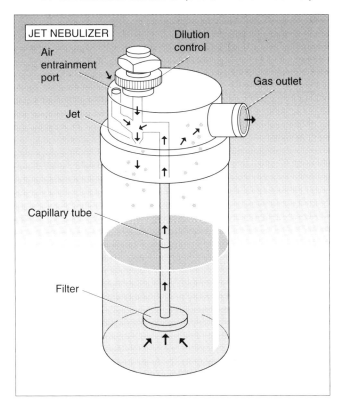

a. Utilizes the Bernoulli principle to draw water up the capillary tube into the gas stream to produce aerosol (mist)
b. Mechanical nebulizers produce about **50%** of their particles in the **0.5- to 3-micron range.**

2. **Hydrosphere (Babington nebulizer)**

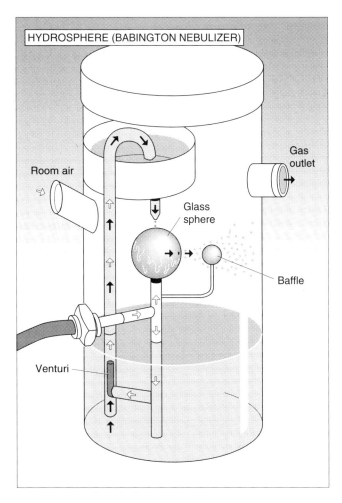

a. Water is pumped up into a reservoir above a glass sphere and drops out of the reservoir onto the sphere. The sphere has a small hole with high-velocity gas coming through it that decreases the pressure, pulling the water over the sphere. Water is then hit by high-velocity gas, producing an aerosol, and the particles hit a baffle, further reducing particle size.
b. Approximately 97% of the aerosol particles produced fall within the 1- to 10-micron range, with 50% smaller than 5 microns.
c. Commonly used to deliver aerosol to an oxygen tent

3. **Small-volume nebulizer** (hand-held nebulizer, medication nebulizer)

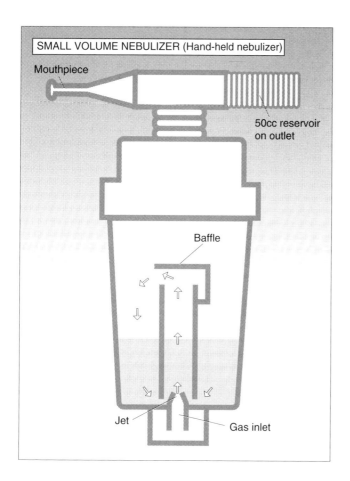

a. Used as a hand-held nebulizer or nebulizer on ventilator or IPPB circuit to deliver medications
b. Usually holds 3 to 6 ml of liquid medication
4. **Metered-Dose Inhaler (MDI)**
   a. This device delivers medication in aerosol form by squeezing the vial, in which the medication is stored, upward into the delivery port. This activates a small valve that allows the pressurized gas to nebulize the medication and deliver it to the patient.
   b. MDIs have become a very popular method for delivering aerosolized drugs to the respiratory tract.
   c. The particle size produced varies from 2 to 40 microns, with only about 10% of the dose actually reaching the lower respiratory tract.
   d. It is essential that the patient be instructed thoroughly and *correctly* on proper use of the MDI to ensure optimal aerosol penetration.

e. The following points on the proper use of the MDI should be emphasized to the patient:
   (1) The patient should be instructed not to place the lips around the delivery port but to keep the mouth opened wide so the teeth and lips will not obstruct the flow of aerosol.
   (2) The MDI should be held about one inch from the mouth, with the delivery port opening directed inside the mouth.
   (3) The patient should be instructed to inhale slowly and as deeply as possible. The MDI should be activated just after the patient has started inhaling.
   (4) Depending on the physician's order, the patient may take two or three aerosol doses in one breath.
   (5) The patient should be instructed to hold the breath at peak inspiration for 5 to 10 seconds for optimal aerosol penetration.
   (6) MDIs are also used in patients on ventilators by placing the device directly into the inspiratory limb of the circuit; it is then activated by the respiratory care practitioner. Ideally, the aerosol should be delivered during a sigh breath with an inspiratory hold.

NOTE: **Spacers and holding chambers, extensions placed on the outlet of the MDI, have proved to be effective in minimizing aerosol loss and increasing the evaporation of the propellant. This increases the stability of the aerosol and results in deeper penetration of the particles.**

F. **Electric nebulizers**
  1. **Impeller nebulizer** (spinning disk or room humidifier)

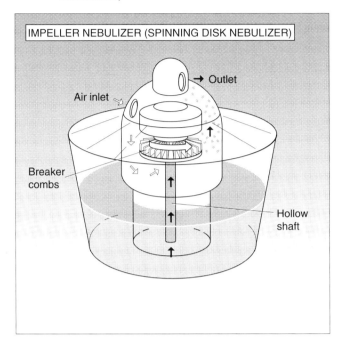

IMPELLER NEBULIZER (SPINNING DISK NEBULIZER)

Outlet
Air inlet
Breaker combs
Hollow shaft

  a. The disk rotates rapidly, drawing water up from the reservoir and throwing it through a slotted baffle, reducing the size of the particles.
  b. Popular for home use but does not produce clinically adequate aerosol output
  c. Difficult to keep clean

2. **Ultrasonic nebulizer**

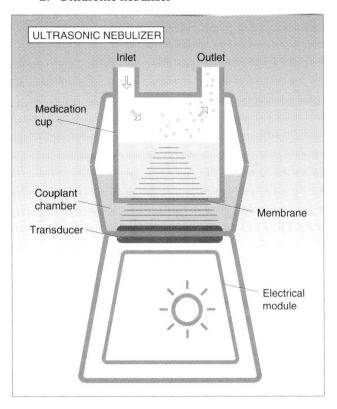

ULTRASONIC NEBULIZER

Inlet
Outlet
Medication cup
Couplant chamber
Transducer
Membrane
Electrical module

  a. A piezoelectric transducer in the couplant chamber of the unit is electrically charged and produces high-frequency vibrations. These vibrations are focused on the diaphragm of the medication cup that sits in the couplant chamber. The vibrations break the medications in the cup into small particles, which are delivered to the patient.
  b. **The frequency** of the electric energy supplied to the transducer is approximately 1.35 megacycles (megacycle = 1 million cycles per second). Some units employ frequency controls that adjust the particle size being delivered to the patient.
  c. The couplant chamber contains cold tap water to help absorb mechanical heat and to act as a transfer medium for the sound waves to the medication cup. Adequate water levels must be maintained in the couplant chamber or mist output from the medication cup will decrease. A couplant chamber indicator light is activated when the water level in the chamber drops to a low level.
  d. **The amplitude control determines the volume of the aerosol output.** Volume may be as high as **6 ml/min**, twice the output of pneumatic nebulizers, **making it the**

nebulizer of choice for patients with thick,
retained sputum.

e. A built-in blower delivers 20 to 30 L/min of
air to the medication cup to aid in aerosol
delivery and help evacuate heat.

f. Ninety percent of the aerosol particles
produced fall within the 0.5- to 3-micron
range.

g. The temperature of the delivery aerosol is
3°C to 10°C above room temperature during
normal operation.

h. Hazards of ultrasonic therapy

(1) Overhydration

(2) Bronchospasm

(3) Sudden mobilization of secretions

(4) Electrical hazard

(5) Water collection in the tubing

(6) Swelling of secretions from the absorp-
tion of saline, obstructing the airway

(7) Changes in drug dosage due to drug
reconcentration as a result of the
evaporation of the solvent in the
medication cup, leading to an increas-
ingly stronger dose as the treatment
continues

G. Important points concerning nebulizers

1. Of all respiratory equipment, heated nebulizers
are the greatest source of delivery of contaminated moisture to the patient, *Pseudomonas*
being the most common contaminant. They
should be replaced every 12 to 24 hours.

2. Make sure that jets and capillary tubes are clear
of debris or build-up of minerals by cleaning
after each use. If the nebulizer is not producing
adequate mist, it could have a clogged capillary
tube or jet.

3. All nebulizers have pressure pop-off valves that
should be checked after the nebulizer is set up
(usually 2 psi). The pop-off will be effective only
if the nebulizer is on 100%.

4. Keep water drained out of the aerosol tubing, as
this will **increase** the delivered oxygen percentage to the patient.

5. Keep the water level at the appropriate markings
on the nebulizer to ensure optimal aerosol
output.

6. Soap should not be used to clean the couplant
chamber or medication cup of the ultrasonic
nebulizer because residue interferes with the
ultrasonic activity. Should interference occur, a
small amount of alcohol in the couplant chamber will help.

7. Make sure the filter at the end of the capillary
tubes of pneumatic nebulizers are decontami-
nated properly. A dirty or clogged filter will not
allow the fluid to be drawn up the tube adequately, reducing aerosol output.

REFERENCES

Eubanks D, Bone R. *Comprehensive Respiratory Care.* 2nd ed.
St. Louis: CV Mosby; 1990.

McPherson SP. *Respiratory Therapy Equipment.* 4th ed. St.
Louis: CV Mosby; 1990.

McPherson SP. *Respiratory Home Care Equipment.* Dubuque,
IA: Kendall/Hunt Publishing; 1988.

Scanlan C, Spearman C. *Egan's Fundamentals of Respiratory
Care.* 5th ed. St. Louis: CV Mosby; 1990.

PRETEST ANSWERS

1. C

2. A

3. D

4. D

5. B

6. C

Equipment Decontamination/ Infection Control

PRETEST QUESTIONS*

1. Which of these devices has the greatest potential for delivering contaminated water to the patient's airway?

A. heated jet nebulizer
B. heated Cascade humidifier
C. bubble humidifier
D. spinning disk nebulizer

2. Which of the following cleaning methods/materials sterilize equipment?

I. pasteurization
II. ethylene oxide gas
III. autoclave
IV. alcohol

A. I only
B. II only
C. II and III only
D. II, III, and IV only

3. What is the most cost-effective method of minimizing the contamination of a tracheostomy patient's airway?

A. Suction every 2 hours using sterile technique.
B. Practice proper handwashing technique.
C. Use disposable equipment.
D. Change the nebulizer every 24 hours.

4. While making oxygen rounds you notice that a disposable nebulizer contains 20 ml of sterile water. What is the appropriate action to take?

A. Let it run until the nebulizer is empty.
B. Refill it with fresh, sterile water.
C. Replace it with a new disposable nebulizer.
D. Pour out the remaining water, rinse with tap water, and add fresh, sterile water.

_____

*See answers at the end of the chapter.

CHAPTER **4**

Equipment Decontamination/ Infection Control

I. BASIC TERMINOLOGY

A. Vegetative organisms — organisms in active growth. **These organisms pose the greatest hazard to respiratory therapy equipment.**

B. Spores — organisms in a resting, resistant stage. They are very difficult to kill, but pose little threat to respiratory therapy equipment.

C. Disinfection — the killing of all vegetative forms of organisms but not spores. Agents that disinfect equipment are called disinfectants.

D. Sterilization — the killing of all organisms, both vegetative and spores. An agent that sterilizes equipment is called a sterilant.

E. -cidal — suffix meaning "to kill" (e.g., **bactericidal** is the killing of bacteria).

F. -static — suffix meaning "to prevent the growth of" (e.g., **bacteriostatic** is preventing the growth of bacteria).

G. Gram-negative organism — an organism that appears red when a Gram's stain test is done. Ex: *Pseudomonas, Klebsiella, Legionella.*

H. Gram-positive organism — an organism that appears blue when a Gram's stain is done. Ex: *Staphylococcus.*

I. Nosocomial infection — a hospital-acquired infection, often caused by *Pseudomonas, Staphylococcus, Candida albicans,* and *Escherichia coli.*

II. CONDITIONS THAT INFLUENCE ANTIMICROBIAL ACTION

A. Chemical concentration — the more concentrated a chemical is, the more rapid the action.

B. Intensity of the physical agent — the more intense a physical agent (heat), the more rapidly the organisms are killed.

C. Time — the longer the organisms are exposed to the agent, the greater the number killed.

D. Temperature — increasing the temperature of a chemical agent shortens the exposure time required to kill the organisms.

E. Type of organism — vegetative forms of bacteria are more easily killed than spore-forming bacteria. Spores are more resistant to both chemical and physical agents.

F. Number of organisms — the more organisms, the longer the exposure time required to kill them.

G. Nature of material bearing the organism — the presence of blood, sputum, and the like provides protection for the organisms. Therefore, **equipment must be thoroughly washed in soapy water and rinsed off prior to the decontamination process.**

III. THREE MAIN CLASSES OF BACTERIA

A. Cocci — spherical-shaped bacteria

B. Spirilla — spiral-shaped bacteria

C. Bacilli — rod-shaped bacteria
   1. Bacilli are the bacteria most frequently found on respiratory equipment.
   2. They **are not** spore-forming bacteria.
   3. Examples of bacilli (frequently responsible for pneumonia):
      a. *Klebsiella pneumoniae* — gram-negative
      b. *Pseudomonas aeruginosa* — gram-negative
      c. *Mycobacterium* — gram-positive (causative agent of tuberculosis)
      d. *Legionella* — gram-negative
      e. *Serratia marcescens* — gram-negative (secondary invader in respiratory and burn patients)
      f. *Haemophilus influenzae* — gram-negative

IV. STERILIZATION AND DISINFECTION TECHNIQUES

A. **Physical agents**
   1. **Moist heat**
      a. Boiling water at 100°C for 5 minutes kills vegetative forms of bacteria, fungi, and most viruses.
      b. Kills organisms by coagulation of the cell protein
      c. Because spores are not killed, this is a disinfection method.
      d. Used mainly at home or in doctors' offices but not recommended for use on respiratory therapy equipment
   2. **Autoclave (steam under pressure)**
      a. Heat in the form of steam is one of the most dependable and practical methods of decontamination.
      b. **Normal operating levels are 15 minutes at 121°C and 15 psig (2 atmospheres).**
      c. **Autoclaving sterilizes equipment.**
      d. Kills organisms by coagulation of the cell protein
      e. Bacteria filters are commonly sterilized by this method, but any material made of rubber cannot withstand the intense heat.
      f. The tops of nebulizers and humidifiers should be attached loosely to allow exposure of all parts of the device.
      g. Equipment to be autoclaved must be thoroughly washed in soapy water, rinsed, dried, and wrapped in muslin, cloth, or a paper bag.
      h. Written on the outside of the wrap should be information including the time and date of processing, what kind of equipment is inside the wrap, and who prepared the equipment for processing.
   3. **Pasteurization**
      a. Equipment must be washed in soapy water and rinsed off prior to placement in the pasteurizing machine.
      b. Equipment is immersed in hot water at 60° to 70°C for 20 to 30 minutes.
      c. The hotter the water, the less time needed to clean the equipment.
      d. **Pasteurization disinfects equipment,** as spores are killed.

B. **Chemical agents**
   1. **Ethylene oxide gas sterilization**
      a. Equipment must be washed in soapy water, rinsed, **dried completely,** and placed in a sealed plastic bag prior to being placed in the sterilization chamber.
      b. If equipment is not completely dry prior to the process, ethylene oxide combines with water to form ethylene glycol, an irritating substance found in antifreeze.
      c. Ethylene oxide kills all organisms including spores; therefore, it **sterilizes equipment.**
      d. It is a highly flammable gas, but the explosive danger may be minimized by mixing it with approximately 90% carbon dioxide or Freon.
      e. Equipment may be processed in one of two ways:
         (1) Warm gas — 50° to 56°C for 4 hours
         (2) Cold gas — 22°C (room temperature) for 6 to 12 hours
      f. After exposure to the gas, the equipment must be aerated for about 12 hours at 50° to 60°C.
      g. Most respiratory therapy equipment can be decontaminated by this method.
      h. The recommended gas concentration is 800 to 1000 mg/L.

i. Because moisture enhances the action of ethylene oxide, the relative humidity within the sterilizing chamber should be maintained at 50% or higher.

j. Items placed in sealed plastic bags are suitable for use for up to 1 year after gas sterilization, provided the bag is intact.

2. **Alcohol**
   a. Ethyl alcohol (95% concentration) and isopropyl alcohol (70% concentration) are the most commonly used alcohols in the clinical setting.
   b. Alcohols are bactericidal and fungicidal but not sporicidal; therefore, they disinfect equipment.
   c. Kills organisms by destroying the cell protein
   d. Action is intensified if mixed with water
   e. Used as a disinfectant to wipe down respiratory therapy equipment

3. **Glutaraldehyde**
   a. Related to formaldehyde
   b. Two types of glutaraldehyde:
      (1) Cidex — alkaline pH (7.8 to 8.5)
      (2) Sonocide — acidic pH (2.7 to 3.7)
   c. These agents are **bactericidal in 10 to 15 minutes and sporicidal in 3 to 10 hours** depending on the temperature of the solution.
   d. Normally used to disinfect equipment but may be used to sterilize
   e. Equipment must be washed in soapy water and rinsed off before placement in the solution bath.
   f. Upon removal from the solution bath (with gloves to prevent irritation), the equipment should be rinsed off and thoroughly dried before packaging.
   g. Kills organisms by coagulation of the cell protein

4. **Acetic acid (vinegar)**
   a. Kills vegetative bacteria but not spores; therefore, it **disinfects equipment.**
   b. **It is very effective against *Pseudomonas.***
   c. Used as a disinfectant for home care equipment and often run through room humidifiers for cleaning purposes
   d. Not recommended for use on respiratory therapy equipment in the clinical setting unless in combination with more effective methods

V. IMPORTANT POINTS CONCERNING DECONTAMINATION OF EQUIPMENT

A. Use only sterile solutions in reservoirs.

B. Solutions left in the reservoir should be discarded before adding fresh solution.

C. Always date the container that holds the solution after it is opened. It should be discarded after 24 hours. This reduces the possibility of filling a reservoir with contaminated solution.

D. Condensation in the delivery tubing **should never be drained back into the reservoir.**

E. Provide a method of routine surveillance to determine the effectiveness of the decontamination process.

F. Use of disposable equipment decreases the potential for cross-contamination. Since warm, moist humidifiers and nebulizers are ideal breeding grounds for bacteria, disposables are for single-patient use only.

G. The most cost-effective method of preventing cross-contamination of equipment is by proper hand-washing techniques.

H. Disposable equipment should not be refilled or reused.

I. Equipment must be completely dry when packaged and stored in order to prevent new growth.

VI. ISOLATION PRECAUTIONS

A. **Respiratory isolation** — prevents the transmission of organisms through direct contact or droplets spread by coughing, sneezing, or breathing.
   1. Handwashing — yes
   2. Gowns — no
   3. Gloves — yes
   4. Masks — yes
   5. Closed doors — yes
   6. Double-bag equipment — yes

B. **Enteric isolation** — prevents the spread of diseases that occur through direct or indirect contact with infected feces or heavily contaminated articles.
   1. Handwashing — yes
   2. Gowns — no
   3. Gloves — yes
   4. Masks — no
   5. Closed doors — no
   6. Double-bag equipment — yes

C. **Strict isolation** — prevents the spread of communicable diseases that can be readily transmitted by both contact and airborne routes.

1. Handwashing — yes
2. Gowns — yes
3. Gloves — yes
4. Masks — yes
5. Closed doors — yes
6. Double-bag equipment — yes

D. **Wound and skin isolation** — prevents the spread of infection through direct contact with heavily contaminated dressings or wounds.

1. Handwashing — yes
2. Gowns — no
3. Gloves — yes
4. Masks — no
5. Closed doors — no
6. Double-bag equipment — no

E. **Reverse isolation** — attempts to prevent the transmission of harmful organisms from hospital personnel or visitors to the infection-prone patient (immunosuppressed patients, cancer or leukopenic patients).

1. Handwashing — yes
2. Gowns — yes
3. Gloves — yes
4. Masks — yes
5. Closed doors — yes
6. Double-bag equipment — no

NOTE: While handwashing is mandatory after contact with every patient, to help prevent the transmission of communicable diseases such as HIV in the hospital setting, other precautions should be taken. *Universal precautions,* the use of gowns, gloves, masks, and protective eyewear, should be followed by practitioners having contact with *all* patients where the exposure to blood or body fluids is possible.

REFERENCES

Barnes TA. *Respiratory Care Practice.* Chicago: Year Book Medical Publishers; 1988.

Eubanks D, Bone R. *Comprehensive Respiratory Care.* 2nd ed. St. Louis: CV Mosby; 1990.

The Merck Manual. 14th ed. Rahway, NJ: Merck and Company; 1982.

PRETEST ANSWERS

1. A

2. C

3. B

4. C

Management of the Airway

PRETEST QUESTIONS*

1. To ensure the proper position of an E-T tube immediately after intubation, the respiratory care practitioner should do which of the following **first**?

A. Obtain a stat chest x-ray.
B. Auscultate the chest while manually ventilating.
C. Measure the length of the tube protruding from the mouth.
D. Observe bilateral chest movement.

2. To maintain an open airway in a comatose patient receiving IPPB therapy, the patient should be positioned

A. in semi-Fowler's position with the neck extended.
B. in reverse Trendelenburg's position.
C. in Trendelenburg's position.
D. on the side with neck flexed.

3. All of the following statements about an oropharyngeal airway are true EXCEPT which of the following?

A. It is tolerated well by alert patients.
B. It should be inserted with the tip toward the roof of the mouth.
C. It should not be taped in place.
D. It may stimulate gagging.

*See answers at the end of the chapter.

4. A patient of average size is orally intubated with an E-T tube that has an internal diameter of 6 mm. After instilling 30 ml of air into the cuff, air is heard coming from the patient's mouth during inspiration. What may be the cause of this problem?

A. Inspiratory flow is too high.
B. There is too much air in the cuff.
C. The E-T tube is in the right main-stem bronchus.
D. The E-T tube is too small relative to the patient's trachea.

5. The purpose of inserting an oropharyngeal airway in an orally intubated ventilator patient is

A. to prevent the tongue from falling back into the oropharynx.
B. to prevent the patient from biting the E-T tube.
C. to facilitate suctioning.
D. to decrease oral secretion production.

6. You have just completed postural drainage and percussion on a patient with no observed side effects. As you begin suctioning the nasopharynx, there is a sudden decrease in heart rate. The most likely cause of this is

A. hypercapnia.
B. hypoxemia.
C. vagal stimulation.
D. coughing.

Management of the Airway

I. UPPER AIRWAY OBSTRUCTION

A. Main causes of upper airway obstruction
1. Tongue falling back against the posterior wall of the pharynx due to unconsciousness or central nervous system (CNS) abnormality.
2. Edema — postextubation inflammation and swelling of glottic area
3. Bleeding
4. Secretions
5. Foreign substances
   a. Foreign bodies
   b. False teeth
   c. Vomitus
6. Laryngospasm

B. Signs of partial upper airway obstruction
1. Crowing, gasping sounds on inspiration
2. Not able to cough (if slight obstruction, patient may be able to cough)
3. Increasing respiratory difficulty
4. Good to poor air exchange (depending on severity of obstruction)
5. Exaggerated chest and abdominal movement without comparable air movement
6. Cyanosis (depending on severity of obstruction)

C. Signs of complete upper airway obstruction
1. Inability to talk
2. Increased respiratory difficulty with no air movement
3. Cyanosis
4. Sternal, intercostal, and epigastric retractions
5. Use of accessory muscles of the neck
6. Extreme panic
7. Unconsciousness and respiratory arrest if obstruction not relieved

D. Treatment of airway obstruction
1. If patients are conscious with a partial airway obstruction, they should be allowed to try to relieve the obstruction themselves.
2. If patients are conscious with a complete airway obstruction due to food or another foreign object, abdominal thrusts must be performed until the object is dislodged (see Chapter 7, "Cardiopulmonary Resuscitation/Manual Resuscitators").
3. If patients are unconscious with a partial or complete airway obstruction most likely caused by the tongue, the head tilt/chin lift will help relieve the obstruction by moving the tongue forward.

II. ARTIFICIAL AIRWAYS

A. Oropharyngeal airway

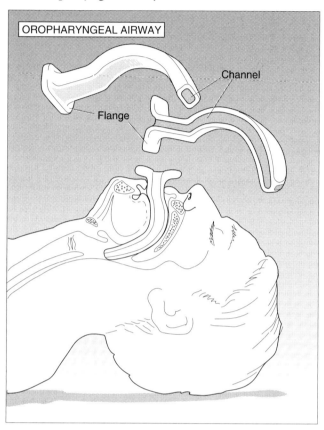

OROPHARYNGEAL AIRWAY

Channel

Flange

1. Maintains a patent airway by lying between the base of the tongue and the posterior wall of the pharynx, preventing the tongue from falling back and occluding the airway
2. **Must only be used on the *unconscious patient,* as a conscious patient would gag on the airway, leading to the potential for aspiration**
3. This airway should **never** be taped in place because a patient regaining consciousness must be able to remove the airway easily to prevent vomiting and aspiration.

4. Proper insertion of the oropharyngeal airway

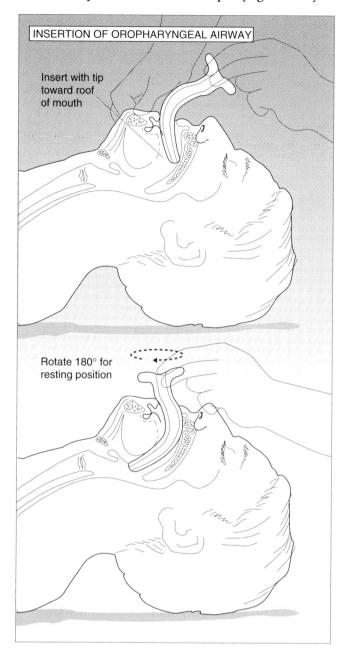

INSERTION OF OROPHARYNGEAL AIRWAY

Insert with tip toward roof of mouth

Rotate 180° for resting position

a. Measure the airway from the corner of the lip to the angle of the jaw to ensure proper length.
b. Remove foreign substances from the mouth.
c. Hyperextend the neck.
d. Using the cross-finger technique, open the patient's mouth and insert the airway with the tip pointing toward the roof of the mouth.
e. Observe the airway passing the uvula and rotate 180°.

5. Hazards of oropharyngeal airways
    a. Gagging or fighting the airway — remove immediately
    b. Base of tongue pushed into the back of the throat, obstructing the airway
    c. Pushing the epiglottis into the laryngeal area with an airway that is too large
    d. Aspiration of the airway or ineffective obstruction relief due to an airway that is too small
6. **Important points concerning oropharyngeal airways**
    a. Oropharyngeal airways may be used in the unconscious, orally intubated patient to prevent the patient from biting the tube.
    b. Berman model airways are made of hard plastic and have a groove down either side to guide a suction catheter to the glottic area.
    c. Guedel model airways are made of a soft, more pliable material and have an opening through the middle to allow the passing of a suction catheter into the glottic area.
B. **Nasopharyngeal airway** (nasal trumpet)

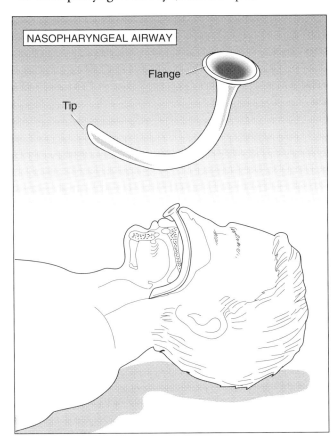

NASOPHARYNGEAL AIRWAY

Flange

Tip

1. Maintains a patent airway by lying between the base of the tongue and the posterior wall of the pharynx

2. Constructed of soft pliable rubber
3. **Proper insertion of the nasopharyngeal airway**
    a. Select the proper size airway by measuring the airway from the tip of the nose to the tragus of the ear. The outside diameter of the airway should be equal to the inside diameter of the patient's internal nares.
    b. Lubricate the airway with a water-soluble gel and insert into patient's nostril.
    c. The flanged end should rest against the nose and the distal tip should rest behind the uvula.
    d. Place tape around the flanged end to secure in place. (May stick safety pin through the flange and tape pin to the face.)
4. This airway is tolerated by the conscious patient.
5. Its primary use is to facilitate nasotracheal suctioning.
6. **Hazards of nasopharyngeal airways**
    a. Aspiration of an airway that is too small
    b. Nasal irritation — alternate nostrils daily
C. **Endotracheal tubes**
    1. **Indications for endotracheal tubes**
        a. Relief of upper airway obstruction — resulting from laryngospasm, epiglottitis, or glottic edema.
        b. Protection of the airway — the airway has four protective reflexes:
            (1) Pharyngeal reflex — gagging and swallowing
            (2) Laryngeal reflex — laryngospasm
            (3) Tracheal reflex — coughing when trachea is irritated
            (4) Carinal reflex — coughing when carina is irritated

NOTE: When these reflexes are obtunded or not functional, the airway must be protected with an E-T tube. These reflexes may be obtunded by paralysis, drugs, loss of consciousness, or neuromuscular disease. As these reflexes become obtunded, they are lost in progression from the pharyngeal to the carinal. As they recover, they do so in progression from the carinal to the pharyngeal.

    c. To facilitate tracheal suctioning
    d. To assist manual or mechanical ventilation
    2. **Hazards of endotracheal tubes**
        a. Contamination of the tracheobronchial tree
        b. Cough mechanism reduced
        c. Damage to the vocal cords
        d. Laryngeal or tracheal edema
        e. Mucosal damage leading to tracheal stenosis
        f. Tube occluded with inspissated secretions

g. Loss of patient's dignity
h. Loss of patient's ability to talk

3. **Steps to perform endotracheal intubation**

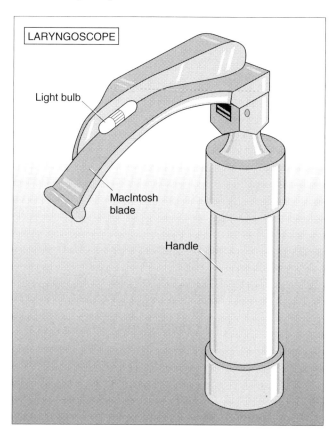

LARYNGOSCOPE

Light bulb

MacIntosh blade

Handle

a. Select a laryngoscope with a **MacIntosh (curved) blade or a Miller (straight) blade.** Make sure the light bulb is tight, as it will not light if loose.

b. Place the patient in the "sniffing position."

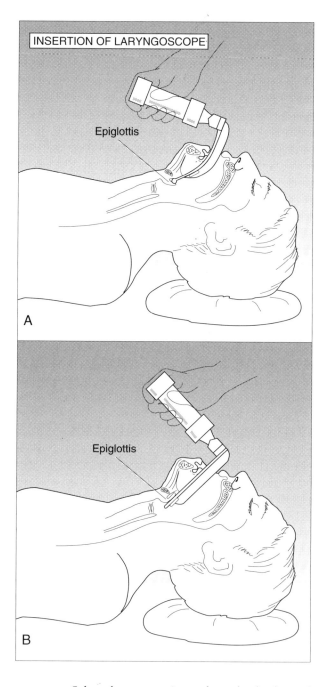

INSERTION OF LARYNGOSCOPE

Epiglottis

A

Epiglottis

B

c. Select the proper size endotracheal tube and insert a stylet to make the tube more rigid for easier insertion. Make sure the stylet does not extend past the end of the tube.

d. Insert the laryngoscope blade into the right side of the mouth (if laryngoscope is in left hand) and move tongue to the left.

e. Advance the blade forward.
   (1) The curved blade (MacIntosh) should be inserted between the epiglottis and the base of the tongue (vallecula), and with a forward and upward motion the epiglottis is raised to expose the glottis and vocal cords.
   (2) The straight blade (Miller) should be placed under the epiglottis and lifted upward and forward to expose the vocal cords.

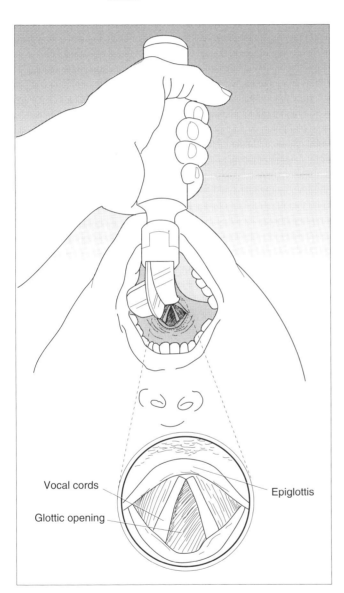

Vocal cords
Glottic opening
Epiglottis

NOTE: Never exceed 15 to 20 seconds per intubation attempt. The blade and tube in the back of the throat may stimulate the vagus nerve, leading to bradycardia. Remove the blade and tube and ventilate with a resuscitator bag and mask. Re-attempt intubation when patient is stabilized.

f. As the vocal cords are observed, advance the E-T tube **approximately 2 inches past the** cords.

NOTE: The average distance from the teeth to the carina is 27 cm. Note that the E-T tube has markings in centimeters indicating the distance to the end of the tube from that point. Therefore, taping the tube at the 23- to 25-cm mark at the teeth will most likely place the tube between the clavicles and the carina.

If the tube is inserted too far, it will enter the right main-stem bronchus.
g. Inflate the cuff and listen for equal and bilateral breath sounds. If louder sounds are heard on the right than on the left, the tube probably is in the right main-stem. Deflate the cuff and withdraw the tube until equal breath sounds are heard.
h. Obtain a stat chest x-ray for tube placement. The end of the tube should rest 2 to 7 cm above the carina. **The carina is located on x-ray at the fourth rib or fourth thoracic vertebra.**
i. Tape the tube securely.

4. **Parts of the endotracheal tube**

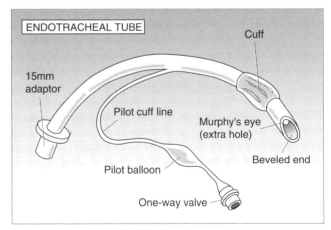

ENDOTRACHEAL TUBE
15mm adaptor
Pilot cuff line
Pilot balloon
One-way valve
Cuff
Murphy's eye (extra hole)
Beveled end

5. **Endotracheal tube markings**
   a. IT (implantation tested) — indicates the material in the tube is nontoxic and free from tissue reaction when implanted in rabbit tissue. (**Polyvinylchloride [PVC] is the most common material used in E-T tubes.**)
   b. Z-79 — the Z-79 Committee for Anesthesia Equipment of the American National Standards Institute. This committee verifies that the tube manufacturer is using material nontoxic to tissues.

c. ID — internal diameter of the tube in millimeters. This is how the tubes are designated by size.

d. OD — outside diameter of the tube in millimeters. Also measured in French units (Fr), equal to one third of a millimeter.

e. Numbers and marks indicating the distance in centimeters from that mark to the distal end of the tube

6. **Complications of oral endotracheal tubes**

a. Poorly tolerated by conscious or semiconscious patients

b. Difficult to stabilize due to tube movement

c. Stimulation of oral secretions

d. Gagging due to tube irritation

e. More difficult to pass suction catheter because of curvature of the tube and poor stabilization

f. Harder to communicate

g. Harder to attach equipment to a poorly stabilized E-T tube

h. Patient may bite the tube, occluding air flow and setting off the high-pressure alarm, thus ending inspiration prematurely.

7. **Nasotracheal tubes**

a. These are considered nonemergency tubes.

b. **Nasotracheal intubation**

(1) Nose should be anesthetized with lidocaine or cocaine spray. A vasoconstrictor such as Neo-Synephrine is used to shrink nasal mucosal blood vessels for easier tube insertion.

(2) Lubricate the tube with water-soluble gel and insert through a patent nostril.

(3) If the patient is alert and breathing spontaneously, try advancing the tube as patient is taking a deep breath or coughing. This is called blind nasal intubation.

(4) If patient is not cooperative or is unconscious, the tube is visualized in the mouth, grasped by **McGill forceps**, and guided through the vocal cords upon direct visualization with a laryngoscope.

(5) Tape the tube in place when proper placement is assured.

c. **Advantages of nasotracheal tubes (versus oral tubes)**

(1) Easier to stabilize

(2) Better tolerated by the patient; gagging is not as likely

(3) Less potential for inadvertent extubation

(4) Equipment attaches more easily

(5) Easier to pass suction catheter

(6) Easier to eat or drink

d. **Complications of nasotracheal tubes**

(1) Pressure necrosis of the nasal tissue

(2) Sinus obstruction leading to sinusitis

(3) Obstruction of eustachian tube, resulting in middle ear infections

(4) Septal deviation

(5) Bleeding during intubation or extubation

D. **Tracheostomy tubes**

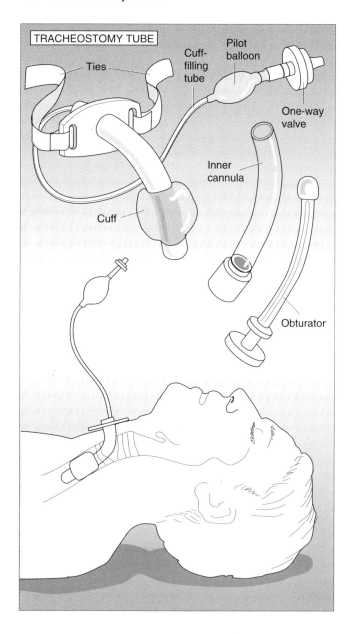

1. Tracheostomy tubes are inserted through an incision (stoma) made between the second and third tracheal rings.

2. The obturator should always be inserted into the outer cannula when the tube is being advanced into the stoma.
3. Once the tube is properly positioned, the obturator should be removed and the inner cannula inserted.
4. The cuff is then inflated and tracheostomy ties are used to secure the tube.
5. Some tubes utilize foam cuffs (Mikity-Wilson Fome Cuff and Kamen Fome Cuff), which are deflated during insertion and allowed to resume normal foam shape when the tube is in place, providing an effective seal against the tracheal wall (exerts low pressure — 20 mm Hg).
6. **Indications for tracheostomies**
   a. Bypass upper airway obstruction
   b. Prevent problems posed by oral or nasal E-T tubes
   c. Allow patient to swallow and receive nourishment
   d. For long-term airway care (E-T tubes should be left in no longer than 3 to 4 weeks)
7. **Immediate complications of tracheostomy tubes** — those occurring within the first 24 hours and associated with the tracheotomy procedure itself
   a. Pneumothorax
   b. Bleeding
   c. Air embolism — tearing of pleural vein
   d. Subcutaneous emphysema
8. **Late complications of tracheostomy tubes** — those occurring more than 1 to 2 days after the tracheotomy
   a. Hemorrhage
   b. Infection
   c. Airway obstruction
   d. Tracheoesophageal fistula
   e. Interference with swallowing

9. **Special tracheostomy tubes**
   a. **Fenestrated tracheostomy tube**

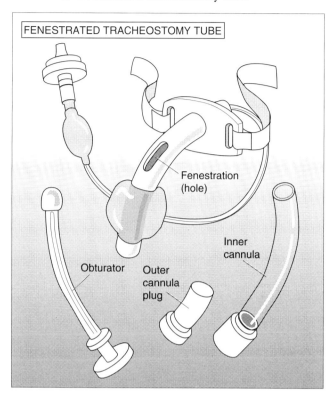

FENESTRATED TRACHEOSTOMY TUBE

Fenestration (hole)

Inner cannula

Obturator

Outer cannula plug

(1) Used to aid in weaning the patient from a tracheostomy tube and allows the patient to talk
(2) With the inner cannula removed, air may pass through the hole (fenestration) in the outer cannula, allowing for weaning from the tracheostomy tube and talking.
(3) The outer cannula may be plugged with the cap on the proximal end of the tube. With the cuff deflated, all air flow will be through the patient's natural airway, but a passage for suctioning will still be available.
(4) Should ventilation be necessary, the inner cannula may be reinserted and the cuff reinflated.

b. **Tracheostomy button**

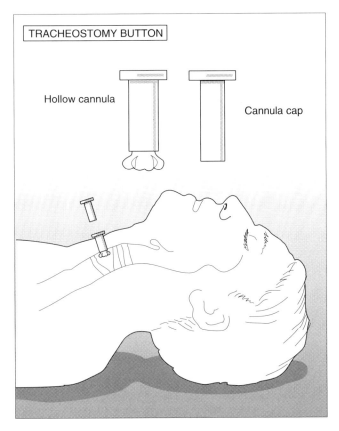

c. **Kistner tracheostomy tube**

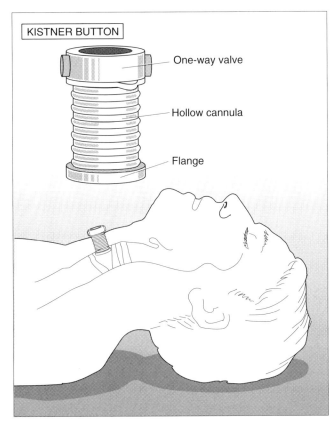

(1) Used to wean the patient from the tracheostomy tube yet maintain a patent stoma

(2) Consists of a short, hollow tube that replaces the tracheostomy tube but maintains the stoma patency should problems arise

(3) The patient has complete use of the upper airway.

(1) Used to wean patient from tracheostomy tube and yet maintain a patent stoma

(2) Kistner tubes are much like tracheostomy buttons except they have a one-way valve on the proximal end of the tube.

(3) Air enters through the one-way valve and the tube during inspiration. As the patient exhales, the valve closes and the air flows up through the vocal cords and out the nose and mouth.

d. **Speaking tracheostomy tubes**

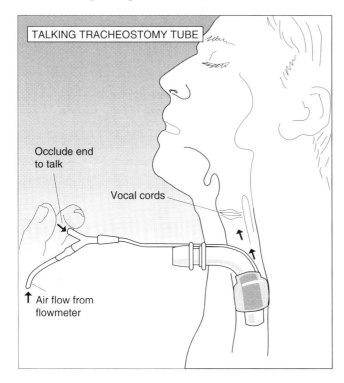

TALKING TRACHEOSTOMY TUBE

Occlude end
to talk

Vocal cords

↑ Air flow from
flowmeter

(1) A constant gas flow is available above
the cuff and around the vocal cords to
allow for speech.

(2) The cuff remains inflated.

III. MAINTENANCE OF ARTIFICIAL AIRWAYS

A. **Cuff care**
 1. Tubes should employ **high-volume, low-
 pressure cuffs only**. These cause less occlusion to
 tracheal blood flow because they apply less
 pressure. They are also called "floppy cuffs." It is
 important to note that if excessive air is placed in
 the cuff it will act as a **high-pressure cuff**.
 2. In order to ensure that the cuff is exerting the
 least amount of pressure on the tracheal wall and
 still providing an adequate seal, **the minimal
 leak technique** or **minimal occluding volume
 technique** should be employed.
 a. With the stethoscope beside the larynx, listen
 for air flow as the cuff is inflated. Inflate the
 cuff until no air flow is heard, then withdraw
 air slowly until a slight leak is heard. **This is
 the minimal leak technique.** (This is often
 performed on a sigh breath from the ventilator.)

b. **The minimal occluding volume technique** is
 accomplished in the same way as the minimal leak technique except the cuff is slowly
 inflated just to the point where no leak is
 heard.
 c. **Cuff pressures should be kept below 20 mm
 Hg if at all possible.**
 d. If the cuff is inflated above 20 mm Hg and a
 leak is still heard, continue inflating the cuff
 using the minimal leak or occluding volume
 technique. It may be the E-T tube is too
 small and more air is needed in the cuff to
 adequately seal the airway. In this case, the
 cuff pressure does not relate to the pressure
 on the tracheal wall.
 e. **Effects of cuff pressure on the tracheal wall**
 (1) Greater than 30 mm Hg — obstructs
 arterial flow resulting in ischemia.
 (2) Greater than 20 mm Hg — obstructs
 venous flow resulting in congestion.
 (3) Greater than 5 mm Hg — obstructs
 lymphatic flow resulting in edema.
B. **Suctioning the airway**
 1. **Technique of suctioning**
 a. Preoxygenate and deep-breathe the patient.
 Hyperoxygenation is preferred to help
 prevent hypoxemia, which may lead to
 bradycardia.
 b. Instill 3 to 5 ml of normal saline to help thin
 secretions (0.3 to 0.5 ml in infants).
 c. Insert the catheter without applying suction
 and advance until an obstruction (carina) is
 met. Do not jab catheter, as this may cause
 bradycardia (vagal stimulation).
 d. Withdraw the catheter approximately 1 to 2
 cm and **apply intermittent suction** while
 rotating the catheter between the thumb and
 finger (**this decreases mucosal damage**).
 e. Never leave the catheter in the airway for
 longer than **15 seconds**.
 f. Upon removal of the catheter, reoxygenate
 and deep-breathe patient and wait 30
 seconds to 1 minute before entering the
 airway again.

**NOTE: Monitor electrocardiogram (EKG)
and stop procedure if complications occur,
hyperoxygenate, and ventilate (if on ventilator).**

g. Repeat steps until secretions are aspirated
 and airway sounds clear.
 2. **Proper suctioning levels**
 a. Adult: –80 to –120 mm Hg

b. Child: –60 to –80 mm Hg
c. Infant: –40 to –60 mm Hg

NOTE: When nasotracheal suctioning is performed, the above steps should be followed in addition to the following techniques:

(1) Lubricate catheter with water-soluble gel.
(2) Instruct patient to take a deep breath or cough as the catheter advances to the oropharynx. This aids in inserting the catheter through the glottic opening.

3. Selecting the proper size catheter
   a. The suction catheter should not occupy more than one half to two thirds of the internal diameter of the tube.

NOTE: If you have a choice of one half or two thirds on the exam, choose one half.

b. Suction catheters are sized by the French unit, **which is equal to 0.33 mm.** Therefore, multiply the catheter size by 0.33 to determine its diameter in millimeters (mm), which is how E-T tubes are sized. To determine the percentage of tube space the catheter occupies, divide the catheter size (mm) by the E-T tube size (mm).

EXAMPLE: How much of the internal diameter of an 8.0-mm E-T tube is occupied by a 14 French suction catheter?

14 French catheter = 4.62 mm (14 **x** 0.33)

$$\frac{4.62 \text{ mm}}{8.0 \text{ mm}} = 0.58 \text{ x } 100 = \mathbf{58\%}$$

4. **Yankauer suction (tonsil)** — used to suction the oropharynx

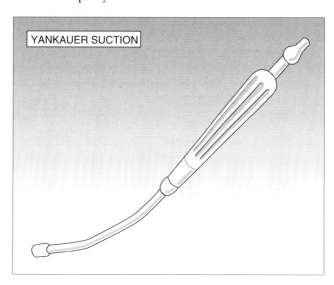

YANKAUER SUCTION

5. **Coudé suction catheter** — angle-tipped catheter used to suction the left lung
6. **Indications for tracheal suctioning**
   a. Remove secretions patient cannot mobilize
   b. Maintain patency of artificial airways
   c. Obtain sputum for culture and sensitivity
7. **Hazards of tracheal suctioning**
   a. Hypoxemia — **increase F_{IO_2} prior to suctioning!**
   b. Arrhythmias — due to hypoxemia and vagal nerve stimulation. **Vagus nerve is stimulated as catheter irritates the oral/nasal mucosa, tracheal mucosa, and carina, causing bradycardia.**
   c. Hypotension — caused by bradycardia and prolonged coughing episode
   d. Atelectasis — caused by using an oversized suction catheter or excessive suction pressure
   e. Tissue trauma — caused by jabbing catheter during insertion, improper lubrication during nasal suction, and not applying **intermittent** suction

IV. ENDOTRACHEAL EXTUBATION

A. **Procedure of extubation**
   1. Explain procedure to the patient.
   2. Increase the F_{IO_2} level.
   3. Suction down the E-T tube.
   4. Suction the mouth and back of throat.
   5. Untape the E-T tube, deflate the cuff, and instruct the patient to take a deep breath. **At peak inspiration, withdraw the tube.**

NOTE: It is permissible to withdraw the tube while suctioning, as this clears the airway while extubating.

B. **Complications of extubation**
   1. **Laryngospasm**
      a. Spasm of the vocal cords due to irritation of the tube, resulting in airway obstruction. Observed by respiratory difficulty immediately following extubation.
      b. If laryngospasm occurs, administer high F_{IO_2} concentration; if it persists for more than 1 to 2 minutes, administer a bronchodilator via a hand-held nebulizer.
   2. **Glottic edema** (see Section V below)

NOTE: Intubation equipment should be readily available at the bedside during extubation should reintubation be necessary.

V. LARYNGEAL AND TRACHEAL COMPLICATIONS OF ENDOTRACHEAL TUBES

A. **Sore throat and hoarseness**
   1. Common occurrence due to tube irritation
   2. Usually subsides within 2 to 3 days
   3. Treat with cool aerosol
B. **Glottic edema**
   1. **Inspiratory stridor** is the major clinical sign.
   2. Caused by:
      a. Traumatic intubation
      b. Insertion of oversized E-T tube
      c. Poor E-T tube maintenance
      d. Allergic response to material in the E-T tube
   3. Treated with:
      a. Cool aerosol to decrease swelling
      b. Vasoconstrictor — racemic epinephrine via hand-held nebulizer
      c. Steroids — dexamethasone occasionally used to reduce swelling
C. **Subglottic edema**
   1. Edema that occurs below the glottis at the level of the cricoid cartilage
   2. A serious complication that occurs following extubation and may lead to reintubation.
   3. If postextubation distress cannot be relieved, subglottic edema must be suspected.
D. **Vocal cord ulceration**
   1. Suspected if hoarseness continues for more than 1 week
   2. Caused by:
      a. Traumatic intubation
      b. Tight-fitting tube
      c. Allergic reaction to material in tube
      d. Excessive tube movement
E. **Tracheal mucosal ulceration**
   1. Common occurrence following extubation
   2. Occurs at the area of the cuff site
F. **Vocal cord paralysis**
   1. Caused by damage to the recurrent laryngeal nerve
   2. Usually occurs secondary to upper chest or neck surgery
G. **Laryngotracheal web**
   1. Caused by necrotic tissue at the glottic or subglottic level that leads to fibrin formation, which combines with secretions and cellular debris to form a membrane or web
   2. If the web breaks loose, it may occlude the airway and result in respiratory distress.
   3. Often occurs several days after extubation
H. **Tracheal stenosis**
   1. A lesion found at the cuff site or the level of the cricoid membrane
   2. As the lesion heals, it constricts, narrowing the airway.
   3. A narrowing of less than 50% of the diameter of the airway will not be symptomatic.
   4. To help prevent tracheal stenosis, maintain cuff pressure by use of the **minimal leak technique.**
I. **Tracheal malacia**
   1. Loss of the cartilaginous support of the trachea
   2. Following extubation, the trachea collapses, leading to respiratory distress.

VI. CHEST PHYSICAL THERAPY

A. These therapies relate to techniques involved in facilitating the clearance of airway secretions and improving the distribution of ventilation by promoting better use of the respiratory muscles. Chest physical therapy (CPT) techniques include the following:
   1. Postural drainage
   2. Chest percussion and vibration
   3. Cough techniques
   4. Breathing exercise training
B. **Goals of chest physical therapy**
   1. Prevent the accumulation of pulmonary secretions
   2. Aid in the mobilization of retained secretions
   3. Improve the distribution of ventilation
   4. Improve cardiopulmonary exercise tolerance

NOTE: An aerosolized bronchodilator via IPPB, hand-held nebulizer, or a metered-dose inhaler should be administered before chest physical therapy. This will aid in alleviating shortness of breath the patient may experience while in the various drainage positions while also improving the mobilization of secretions from the airway.

C. Indications for chest physical therapy
   1. Acute conditions with copious amounts of secretions
      a. Cystic fibrosis
      b. Lung abscess
      c. Pneumonia
      d. Bronchiectasis
   2. Acute respiratory failure with the presence of retained secretions

3. Acute atelectasis
4. Ventilation/perfusion abnormalities resulting from retained secretions
5. COPD patients with inefficient breathing patterns
6. Preventive use for postoperative respiratory complications

D. **Postural drainage positions**

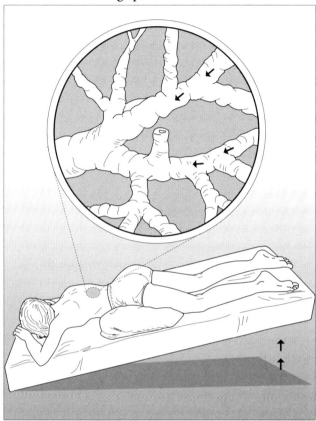

Position to drain the posterior basal segment of the lower lobe

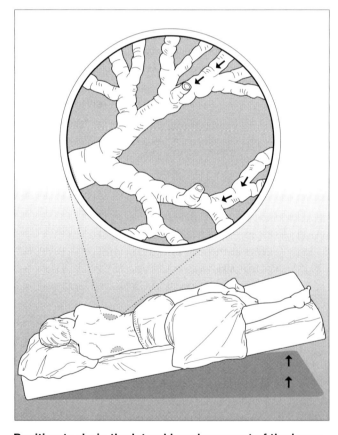

Position to drain the lateral basal segment of the lower lobe

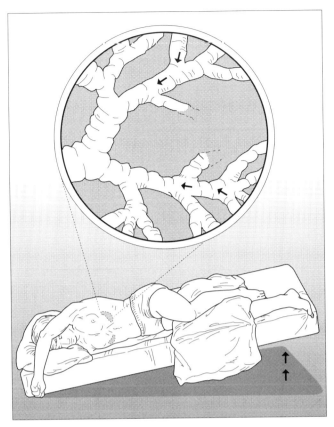

Position to drain the anterior basal segment of the lower lobe

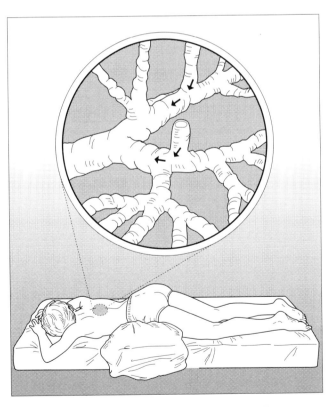

Position to drain the superior segment of the lower lobe

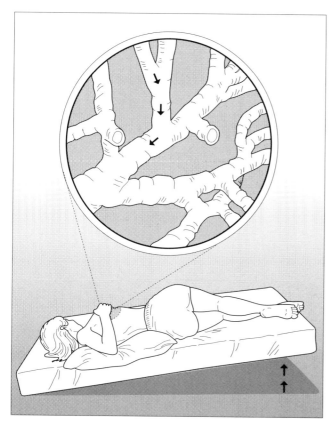

Position to drain the lateral and medial segments of the middle lobe

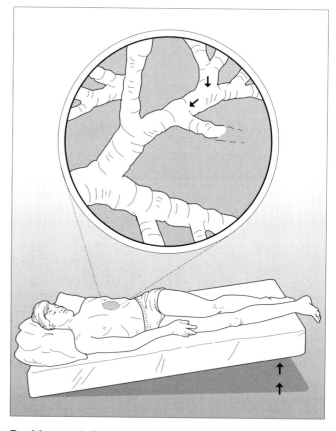

Position to drain the superior and inferior lingular segments

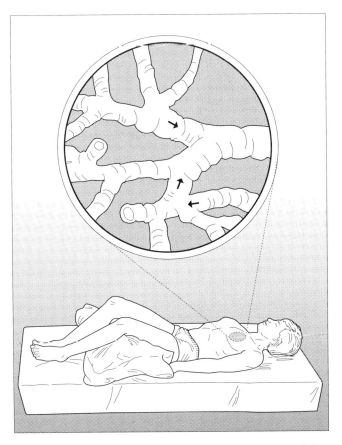

Position to drain the anterior segment of the upper lobe

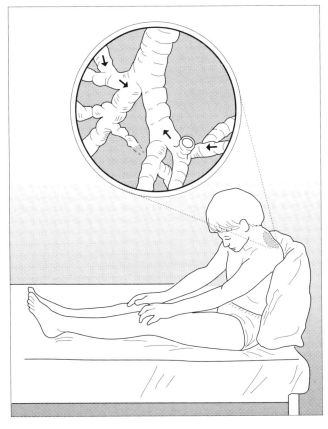

Position to drain the apical segment of the upper lobe

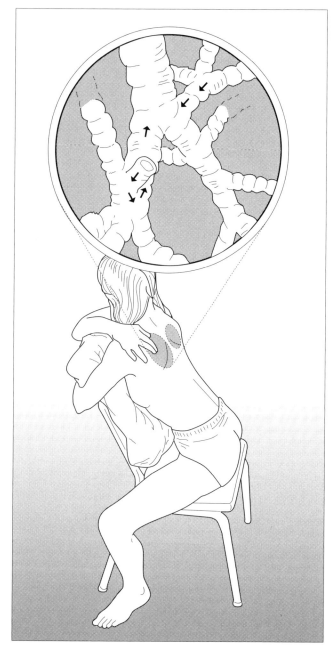

Position to drain the posterior segment of the upper lobe

E. Contraindications for postural drainage
1. Unstable head and neck injury
2. Spinal injury or recent spinal surgery
3. Intracranial pressure >20 mm Hg
4. Hemoptysis
5. Hemorrhage
6. Hemodynamic instability
7. Pulmonary edema associated with congestive heart failure
8. Large pleural effusion
9. Rib fracture
10. Pulmonary embolism
F. **Percussion**
1. Almost always used in conjunction with postural drainage
2. Manual percussion is performed by striking the patient's chest with a cupped hand. A hollow sound should be heard, with secretions loosening from the airways and mobilizing up the tracheobronchial tree.
3. Mechanical vibrators/percussors are commonly used and are more effective than manual percussion because a continuous energy wave is transmitted through the chest wall, improving the mobilization of secretions.
4. Percussion should never be performed over:
a. Clavicles
b. Scapulae
c. Sternum
d. Spine
e. Female breasts
G. **Vibration**
1. Manual vibration should be performed on **exhalation only** after the patient has taken a deep breath. The practitioner applies slight to moderate pressure manually or with a mechanical vibrator over the affected lung segment.
2. Aids in the mobilization of secretions
H. **Adverse effects of chest physical therapy**
1. Hypoxemia
a. Especially in COPD, cardiac, and obese patients
b. May be minimized by delivery of bronchodilator prior to treatment and supplemental oxygen and by modifying drainage positions (omit Trendelenburg position if not tolerated)
2. Rib fractures
3. Increased airway resistance
4. Increased intracranial pressure
a. Avoid Trendelenburg's position in head trauma patients.
b. Coughing results in elevated ICP.

5. Hemorrhage
6. Impaired cardiac output
7. Vomiting with aspiration (withhold CPT until at least 1 hour following meals)

NOTE: Respiratory rate, heart rate, and blood pressure should be monitored before, during, and after CPT.

I. **Cough technique**
  1. While in a sitting position, the patient should inhale through the nose and hold breath for 3 to 5 seconds.
  2. Clasp arms across the abdomen and produce three sharp coughs without taking a breath and while pressing the arms into the abdomen.
  3. Use a pillow to splint thoracic or abdominal incisions to decrease pain and improve the cough effort.

J. **Breathing exercises**
  1. **Pursed-lip breathing**
    a. Should be taught to patients who experience premature airway closure
    b. Patient should be instructed to inhale through the nose and exhale through pursed lips
    c. Helps patient gain control of dyspnea
    d. Provides improved ventilation prior to a cough effort
    e. Teaches patient better control of rate and depth of breathing
    f. Prevents premature airway collapse by generating a back pressure into the airways
    g. Has psychological benefits
  2. **Diaphragmatic breathing**
    a. Teaches the COPD patient to use the diaphragm rather than accessory muscles during breathing
    b. The patient or respiratory care practitioner places a hand over the abdomen as the patient, lying supine, concentrates on moving the hand upward on inspiration. (A book or weight may be substituted for a hand.)

  c. Increased use of the diaphragm will result in a decreased respiratory rate, increased tidal volume, decreased FRC, and increased ventilation
  3. **Segmental breathing**
    a. Similar to diaphragmatic breathing exercise except hand is placed over a specific lung area with atelectasis, secretions, or decreased air flow
    b. The patient should concentrate on moving the hand outward on inspiration.

REFERENCES

Eubanks D, Bone R. *Comprehensive Respiratory Care.* 2nd ed. St. Louis: CV Mosby; 1990.

McPherson SP. *Respiratory Therapy Equipment.* 4th ed. St. Louis: CV Mosby; 1990.

Scanlan C, Spearman C. *Egan's Fundamentals of Respiratory Care.* 5th ed. St. Louis: CV Mosby; 1990.

Shapiro B. *Clinical Application of Respiratory Care.* 4th ed. St. Louis: Mosby Year Book Publishers; 1990.

PRETEST ANSWERS

1. B
2. A
3. A
4. D
5. B
6. C

CHAPTER **6**

Intermittent Positive Pressure Breathing (IPPB) Therapy/Incentive Spirometry

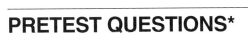

PRETEST QUESTIONS*

1. Which of the following will increase the delivered tidal volume to a patient taking an IPPB treatment with the Bird Mark 7?

  I. Increasing the pressure
 II. Increasing the flow
III. Increasing the sensitivity
IV. Decreasing the flow

  A. I only
  B. I and II only
  C. I and IV only
  D. II and III only

2. While IPPB is being administered, the patient complains of feeling dizzy and lightheaded. What should the respiratory care practitioner do to correct this?

  A. Increase the pressure.
  B. Have the patient pause longer between breaths.
  C. Decrease the sensitivity.
  D. Instruct the patient to breathe faster.

3. While IPPB is being administered, the patient's heart rate increases from 86 to 115 beats/min. The appropriate action is to

  A. continue the treatment but observe closely.
  B. stop the treatment and notify the physician.
  C. decrease inspiratory pressure.
  D. allow the patient a 5-minute rest, then resume therapy.

4. During an IPPB treatment, the patient suddenly complains of chest pain and becomes short of breath. Upon assessing the patient, you auscultate decreased breath sounds on the left and the trachea is shifted to the right. These findings are consistent with

  A. right-sided pneumothorax.
  B. atelectasis of the left lung.
  C. pleural effusion.
  D. left-sided tension pneumothorax.

5. While taking an IPPB treatment, the patient complains he or she can't cycle the machine off. Which of the following could be causing this?

  I. Sensitivity is set too low
 II. Not enough air in E-T tube cuff
III. Malfunction of exhalation valve
IV. Leak around medication nebulizer
  A. I only
  B. I and II only
  C. III and IV only
  D. II, III, and IV only

6. Which of the following is not necessary for incentive spirometry to be effective?

  A. Cooperative patient
  B. Respiratory rate <12
  C. Motivated patient
  D. FVC >15 ml/kg of body weight

---

*See answers at the end of the chapter.

CHAPTER **6**

Intermittent Positive Pressure Breathing (IPPB) Therapy/ Incentive Spirometry

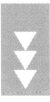

I. INTRODUCTION TO INTERMITTENT POSITIVE PRESSURE BREATHING (IPPB) THERAPY

A. Intermittent positive pressure breathing is defined as a short-term (10 to 15 min) breathing treatment in which above atmospheric pressures are delivered to the patient's lungs via a pressure-limited ventilator.

B. Effective IPPB is dependent on four factors:
1. A respiratory care practitioner who has been well trained and exhibits a knowledge of the equipment, medications delivered, reasons for therapy, side effects of therapy, and goals of therapy
2. A relaxed, informed, and cooperative patient
3. A pressure-limited IPPB machine with a means of measuring tidal volume
4. Proper practitioner instruction on breathing patterns and cough techniques

II. PHYSIOLOGIC EFFECTS OF IPPB

A. **Increased mean airway pressure**
1. During normal spontaneous inspiration, airway pressure drops below atmospheric pressure (-2 cm H_2O), thereby setting up a pressure gradient between the atmosphere (at nose and mouth) and the airways. Air flows into the airways, gradually building pressure back up to the atmospheric level. Air flow stops and passive exhalation occurs due to natural recoil properties of lung tissue. The lung is never subjected to significant positive pressure.
2. During an IPPB machine breath, positive pressure is applied to the airways to improve the ventilation status of the lung. This is what is meant by **increased mean airway pressure**. It is the average (mean) pressure in the airways during one breathing cycle.

B. **Increased tidal volume**
1. IPPB should deliver tidal volumes of 12 to 15 ml/kg of ideal body weight.

2. Delivered tidal volume (V_T) is dependent on the patient's lung status (compliance, airway resistance, etc.).
   a. Decreased compliance — decreased delivered tidal volume
   b. Increased compliance — increased delivered tidal volume
   c. Decreased airway resistance — increased delivered tidal volume
   d. Increased airway resistance — decreased delivered tidal volume
3. Exhaled tidal volume may be measured with the use of a respirometer or gas collection bag on the exhalation port.
4. The inspiratory pressure control adjusts the delivered tidal volume.
   a. Increase pressure — increase delivered tidal volume
   b. Decrease pressure — decrease delivered tidal volume

C. **Decreased work of breathing**
   1. A patient experiencing acute hypoventilation may avoid intubation and placement on mechanical ventilation by administration of frequent IPPB treatments (may be temporary).
   2. The practitioner must encourage the patient to relax and allow the IPPB unit to do all the work in order for the patient's work of breathing to decrease.
   3. IPPB may increase the patient's work of breathing if:
      a. The machine sensitivity is set too low, making it difficult for the patient to cycle the machine into inspiration. **The patient should pull no more than –2 cm H$_2$O pressure to initiate inspiration.**
      b. The flowrate is inadequate to meet the patient's inspiratory flow demands. Increase the flowrate if inspiratory time is prolonged and the manometer needle **rises slowly** to peak pressure.
      c. The delivered tidal volume is inadequate. Monitor tidal volume and listen to basilar breath sounds to ensure adequate volumes are being delivered.
      d. Adequate time is not allowed for passive exhalation to occur. The machine **sensitivity** may be set **too high** causing inspiration to begin prematurely.

D. **Alteration of the inspiratory (I) and expiratory (E) pattern**
   1. Placing a patient with respiratory difficulties on IPPB should improve alveolar ventilation, thereby making the patient more comfortable

and less "air hungry" and returning the I/E times and respiratory rate to normal.
   2. Normal I:E ratio for an adult is 1:2.

E. **Mechanical bronchodilation**
   1. A patient with respiratory disease will experience an increased resistance to air flow as the diameter of the airways decreases due to bronchospasm, secretions, and other factors.
   2. When positive pressure is applied to constricted airways, dilation of these airways can occur to a greater degree than with spontaneous breathing.

NOTE Some studies show that higher flowrates and pressures may cause a bronchoconstrictive reflex in the airways. This may be counteracted by the use of bronchodilators.

F. **Cerebral function**
   1. A patient being administered IPPB may experience lightheadedness, dizziness, or faintness due to reduced Pa$_{CO_2}$ levels and resultant alkalemia. **Decreased Pa$_{CO_2}$ levels result in cerebral vasoconstriction and decreased cerebral blood flow.**
   2. In order to prevent reduced Pa$_{CO_2}$ levels, encourage the patient to breathe slowly and to pause between breaths.
   3. A 50-ml flex tube should be connected between the mouthpiece and manifold to allow for a slight rebreathing of carbon dioxide, preventing decreased Pa$_{CO_2}$ levels.

III. INDICATIONS FOR IPPB THERAPY

A. Increased work of breathing
B. Hypoventilation
C. Inadequate cough
D. Increased airway resistance
E. Atelectasis — especially sedated postoperative patients
F. Pulmonary edema
G. Aid in weaning from continuous mechanical ventilation
H. Placebo effect

IV. HAZARDS OF IPPB THERAPY

A. **Excessive ventilation**
   1. Leads to decreased Pa$_{CO_2}$ levels, causing cerebral vasoconstriction and resultant dizziness

2. Patient should be instructed not to walk immediately following the treatment

B. **Excessive oxygenation**
   1. Patients with moderate to severe COPD breathe because of the "hypoxic drive" mechanism. If the IPPB treatment is given with oxygen, it may elevate the Pa_{O_2} above the patient's normal level (50 to 60 torr), knocking out the drive to breathe (see Chapter 10, "Lung Disorders").
   2. Hypoxic drive potential should be noted with the following arterial blood-gas values:
      a. pH — 7.35 to 7.40 (compensated)
      b. Pa_{CO_2} — >50 torr
      c. Pa_{O_2} — <60 torr
      d. HCO_3 — >30 mEq/L

C. **Decreased cardiac output**
   1. Positive pressure applied to the airways will also be exerted on blood vessels returning blood to the heart. This restricts venous blood return to the heart, which in turn decreases cardiac output from the left ventricle.
   2. Avoiding high inspiratory pressures and long inspiratory times will minimize this hazard.
   3. If there is a decreased venous return during the therapy, the patient may experience **tachycardia** due to decreased left ventricular filling pressure, as well as a **drop in systemic blood pressure.**

D. **Increased intracranial pressure**
   1. Blood flow from the head is restricted as positive pressure is exerted on the superior vena cava returning blood to the heart. This keeps more blood in the cerebral vessels, elevating ICP levels.
   2. Normal ICP level is <10 mm Hg.
   3. Lower pressures and shorter inspiratory times (increased flows) and having the patient in the Fowler's position or sitting on the edge of the bed will minimize this hazard.
   4. This is not a common hazard except in patients with closed head injuries or CNS disease.

E. **Pneumothorax**
   1. Most common in COPD patients with bullous disease or emphysema with bleb formation
   2. Patient complaining of sudden chest pain, shortness of breath, or other breathing difficulties and tachycardia during IPPB must be suspected of having a pneumothorax.
   3. Listen with stethoscope for bilateral breath sounds and observe for asymmetrical chest movement.
   4. **If pneumothorax is suspected, treatment must be stopped immediately.**

F. **Hemoptysis**
   1. Coughing up blood during or after IPPB may not be caused by IPPB itself but may be related to a strong cough accompanying the treatment.
   2. Treatment must be stopped immediately, as air could be forced into a blood vessel and cause an air embolism.

G. **Gastric distention**
   1. Caused by swallowing air during the treatment
   2. May cause the patient to complain of nausea during or after the treatment

H. **Nosocomial infection**
   1. Circuits should be changed every 24 hours.
   2. Appropriate filters should be utilized on the IPPB unit to prevent machine contamination.
   3. The practitioner should wash hands before and after every treatment.

V. CONTRAINDICATIONS FOR IPPB THERAPY

A. **Untreated pneumothorax**
   1. This is considered an **absolute contraindication.** IPPB should not be administered under any circumstances with this condition as it will only worsen the problem.
   2. IPPB is safe for patients with a pneumothorax with a chest tube in place.

B. **Pulmonary hemorrhage**
   1. This is considered an **absolute contraindication.**
   2. If IPPB is administered in this situation, air may enter a blood vessel, resulting in an air embolism.

The following are **relative contraindications**, indicating that IPPB may be administered under certain circumstances.

C. **Tuberculosis**
   1. IPPB may lead to the spread of tuberculosis if patient is not receiving antituberculosis medications.
   2. IPPB is safe if patient is receiving antituberculosis drugs.

D. **Subcutaneous emphysema**
   1. Indicates an air leak from the lung. Further positive pressure would worsen the condition.
   2. Subcutaneous emphysema is not a danger in itself but may indicate a more severe condition such as a pneumothorax or pneumomediastinum.

E. **Hemoptysis**
   1. This condition indicates an open pulmonary blood vessel that could lead to an air embolism.
   2. The origin of the bleeding must be determined.

F. **Closed head injury**
   1. IPPB may increase ICP; therefore, it must be monitored closely in this type of patient.

2. To lessen the potential for increased ICP, use <u>higher flowrates (decreased inspiratory time) and lower peak pressures.</u>

G. **Bullous disease**
   1. Patients with bullae or bleb formation (e.g., COPD patients) are more prone to a pneumothorax, as the weak areas of the lung may rupture.
   2. Use of lower peak inspiratory pressures helps alleviate this problem.
   3. Rupturing of blebs or bullae may result from a strong cough effort during the treatment. These patients must be monitored closely.

H. **Cardiac insufficiency**
   1. Patients with decreased blood pressure, decreased cardiac output, or other such cardiac problems must be monitored closely for further cardiac embarrassment.
   2. Further cardiac problems may result from the positive pressure causing decreased venous return or from cardiac side effects caused by the administered bronchodilator.

I. **COPD patient with air trapping**
   1. IPPB may lead to an increase in air trapping in these patients, causing an inadvertent PEEP that may decrease cardiac output.
   2. IPPB could lead to a further hyperinflated lung status, compromising adequate ventilation.

J. **Uncooperative patient**
   1. Patient must be cooperative for therapy to be effective.
   2. Alternative therapy should be considered.

VI. IPPB IN THE TREATMENT OF PULMONARY EDEMA

A. **IPPB aids in the treatment of pulmonary edema by:**
   1. Decreasing venous return.
   2. Increasing tidal volume to improve ventilation and oxygenation, resulting in improved cardiac activity.
   3. Reducing the alveolar-capillary pressure gradient, thereby reducing the amount of fluid pouring into the airways from the capillaries.
   4. Delivering aerosolized ethanol (40% to 50%), which results in the dissipation of foamy edema fluid.

B. **Other treatments for pulmonary edema**
   1. Diuretics

   2. Cardiac glycosides to improve contractility of the heart and increase cardiac output
   3. Oxygen therapy

VII. PROPER ADMINISTRATION OF IPPB

A. Assemble all equipment and check machine for leaks.
B. Affirm physician order — **If there is some question about the order, such as medication dosage, contact the physician for clarification.**
C. Briefly review patient chart.
   1. Last treatment given
   2. Latest chest x-ray interpretation
   3. Latest arterial blood gas (ABG) results
D. Wash hands.
E. Identify patient by wristband, introduce yourself, and explain the reasons for administering the treatment.
F. Connect the circuit to the IPPB unit and plug into gas source.
G. Place medications in nebulizer.
H. Auscultate breath sounds to locate problem areas (atelectasis, secretions, etc.).
I. Determine heart rate and respiratory rate.
J. Position patient in an upright position for better ventilation.
K. Place the mouthpiece in patient's mouth and encourage patient to keep lips sealed tight and breathe only through the mouth. (Use noseclips if patient has difficulty doing this.)

NOTE: Patients having difficulty keeping their lips sealed tightly around the mouthpiece (leading to leaks and the inability of the IPPB unit to cycle into expiration) should have the treatment altered by using a sealed mouthpiece or mask in place of the mouthpiece.

L. Instruct patient to "sip" on the mouthpiece and allow the machine to fill the lungs until it cycles off. Patient should **hold breath for a count of three prior to exhalation** to better distribute medications and improve gas exchange. Instruct patient to **pause before the next breath.**
M. Set machine parameters.
   1. Inspiratory pressure — Start at lower than desired pressure and gradually increase as therapy continues. As the pressure is increased, likewise increase the flow. This will maintain a fairly constant inspiratory time.

2. Flowrate
3. Nebulization
4. Sensitivity

N. Check vital signs halfway through the treatment. Allow for a brief rest period.

NOTE: If the pulse rate increases by more than 20 beats/min, stop treatment and notify the physician.

O. After 10 minutes or after the medications are completely nebulized, encourage the patient to cough.
P. Check vital signs again.
Q. Encourage patient to cough periodically for the next 30 minutes to 2 hours, as the peak effect of the medications occurs during this time.
R. Wash hands.
S. Record vital signs, tolerance to treatment, cough effort, and sputum characteristics (color, amount, consistency) on the patient's chart.

VIII. CHARACTERISTICS OF SPECIFIC IPPB UNITS

A. **Bird Mark 7**
   1. The Bird Mark 7 is a pneumatically powered

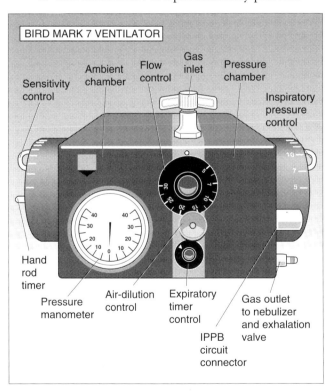

and controlled ventilator. It is designed to operate with oxygen or air at a pressure of 50 psi. It is pressure limited and may be cycled on by patient, by time, or manually.

2. **Gas flow through the Bird Mark 7**
   a. Gas enters the unit from the 50-psig wall outlet through a brass filter.
   b. Gas first travels to the **flowrate control**, a simple needle valve.
   c. From the flowrate control, gas travels to the **ceramic switch** positioned between the ambient chamber and pressure chamber of the unit. Depending on the position of the ceramic switch, flow is either blocked or allowed through.
   d. Patients can cycle the unit into inspiration by creating enough negative pressure to separate a metal clutch plate from a magnet in the ambient chamber. This pulls the ceramic switch to the right, allowing gas flow to continue through the unit.
   e. Gas flow splits as it passes the ceramic switch, with part of the flow supplying the expiratory drive line and nebulizer and the other part flowing into the ambient chamber then through a venturi that entrains ambient air. This increases flow and decreases oxygen percentage.
   f. The "mixed" gas now travels through the venturi gate and into the pressure chamber where the patient circuit is connected and flow continues on to the patient.
   g. Inspiration ends as gas in the patient's lungs builds to a pressure that overcomes the magnetic force between another magnet and metal clutch plate located in the pressure chamber.

3. **Bird Mark 7 controls**
   a. **Flowrate control**
      (1) The scale numbers are simply reference numbers and do not represent liters per minute.
      (2) Flows available are 0 to 80 L/min on air mix and 0 to 50 L/min on 100%.
      (3) Increase flow — decrease inspiratory time
          Decrease flow — increase inspiratory time
      (4) Flow-wave patterns on Bird Mark 7
          (a) Square wave (constant flow) on 100%

(b) Tapered wave (decelerating flow) on air mix

b. **Air mix control**
(1) When pulled out, it allows flow into the ambient chamber and through a Venturi, resulting in air entrainment and oxygen percentage of 40% to 90%.
(2) When pushed in, it blocks the flow to the ambient chamber, eliminating air entrainment and delivering 100% oxygen.
(3) Air mix — higher flowrates
100% oxygen — lower flowrates

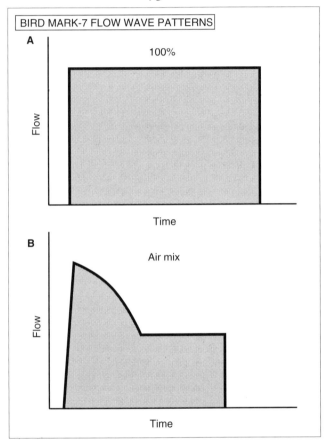

BIRD MARK-7 FLOW WAVE PATTERNS

c. **Inspiratory pressure control**
(1) Adjusts the position of the magnet in the pressure chamber relative to the metal clutch plate
(2) The closer the magnet is to the metal clutch plate, the higher the inspiratory pressure required to move the clutch plate and vice versa.
(3) Increase pressure — increase tidal volume
Decrease pressure — decrease tidal volume

d. **Sensitivity control**
(1) Adjusts the position of the magnet in the ambient chamber relative to the metal clutch plate
(2) The closer the magnet is to the metal clutch plate, the more negative pressure is required by the patient to cycle the machine into inspiration and vice versa.
(3) The magnet should be positioned so that the patient need not generate more than -2 cm H_2O pressure to initiate inspiration.

e. **Expiratory timing device**
(1) A needle valve that controls a leak from the expiratory timer cartridge and used to automatically cycle the unit
(2) Should always be turned off while administering IPPB or unit will self-cycle

f. **Hand timer rod**
(1) Located on the left side of the unit (ambient pressure side) and used to manually cycle the unit off or on

B. **Bennett PR-2 ventilator**

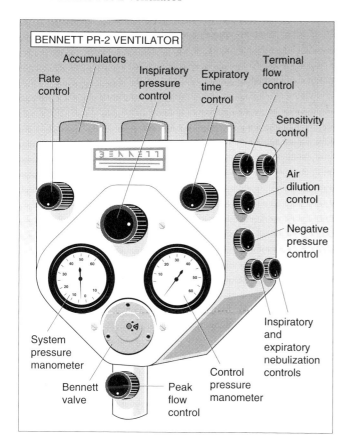

1. The PR-2 is a pneumatically powered, pressure-limited ventilator that may be patient- or time-cycled and time-limited.
2. **Diluter regulator**
   a. An adjustable reducing valve that controls the pressure generated in the patient circuit
   b. Adjustable from 0 to 50 cm H_2O
3. **Bennett valve**
   a. This is the heart of the PR-2. Gas flows from the diluter regulator to this valve and rotates it to the opened position. Gas then travels on to the patient via the circuit. Valve also opens in response to patient's negative pressure.
   b. As inspiratory pressure increases, the flow begins to decrease (due to decreased pressure gradient). This rotates the Bennett valve to the closed position, stopping gas flow.
   c. When inspiratory flow decreases to 1 to 4 L/min, the valve will rotate to the off position, stopping gas flow and ending inspiration.
4. **PR-2 controls**

a. **Inspiratory pressure control**
   (1) Adjusts the peak inspiratory pressure
   (2) Adjustable from approximately 0 to 50 cm H_2O
b. **Dilution control**
   (1) When dilution control is pushed in, air entrainment occurs and delivered oxygen percentage varies from 40% to 90%.
   (2) When control is pulled out, no air entrainment is allowed and 100% oxygen is delivered.
c. **Terminal flow control**
   (1) Provides an additional 12 to 15 L/min of flow below the Bennett valve to help cycle the unit off in case leaks are present
   (2) This added flow goes to a venturi that decreases the oxygen percentage (especially important if patient is on 100% oxygen).
d. **Sensitivity control**
   (1) Turning control counterclockwise increases the sensitivity, making it easier for the patient to cycle the unit into inspiration and vice versa.
   (2) When the sensitivity is turned off, it is factory set for the patient to initiate inspiration by generating –0.5 cm H_2O pressure.
e. **Peak flow control**
   (1) In full open position (all the way to the left), the flow is approximately 90 to 100 L/min with air dilution and 20 cm H_2O pressure.
   (2) In full closed position (all the way to the right), the flow is approximately 15 L/min.
f. **Nebulization control**
   (1) Separate controls for inspiratory or expiratory nebulization
   (2) Gas sent to the nebulizer is source gas (100% if plugged into oxygen outlet); therefore, oxygen percentage increases when nebulizing medications.
g. **Rate control and expiratory time**
   (1) Used to automatically cycle the unit on
   (2) Turning rate control to the right sets the rate (adjustable from 0 to 50 breaths/min).
   (3) Expiratory time control lengthens expiratory time.
   (4) These controls should be turned off during the administration of IPPB or the unit will self-cycle.

IX. IMPORTANT FACTORS TO CONSIDER WHEN VENTILATING A PATIENT WITH A PRESSURE-LIMITED IPPB MACHINE

A. Effects on delivered tidal volume
  1. Increased airway resistance — decreased tidal volume
  2. Decreased airway resistance — increased tidal volume
  3. Increased lung compliance — increased tidal volume
  4. Decreased lung compliance — decreased tidal volume
  5. Increased inspiratory pressure — increased tidal volume
  6. Decreased inspiratory pressure — decreased tidal volume
  7. Increased flowrate — decreased tidal volume
  8. Decreased flowrate — increased tidal volume
B. Effects on inspiratory time
  1. Increased flowrate — decreased inspiratory time
  2. Decreased flowrate — increased inspiratory time
  3. Increased lung compliance — increased inspiratory time
  4. Decreased lung compliance — decreased inspiratory time
  5. Increased airway resistance — decreased inspiratory time
  6. Decreased airway resistance — increased inspiratory time

X. PROBLEMS ENCOUNTERED IN ADMINISTERING IPPB AND CORRECTIVE ACTIONS

A. The patient is having difficulty cycling the IPPB machine into the inspiratory phase.
  1. Corrective actions:
    a. Adjust the sensitivity so that the patient has to generate –0.5 to –2 cm H_2O pressure to start inspiration.
    b. Make sure machine is plugged into wall gas outlet.
    c. Ensure machine tubing connections are all tight.
    d. Ensure the patient has lips sealed tightly around the mouthpiece; if a mask is used, ensure that there are no leaks around it.
    e. If the Bird Mark 7 is used, ensure the flow control is turned on.
B. The patient complains of dizziness and tingling in the extremities during the treatment, with no appreciable increase in heart rate.
  1. Corrective action:
    a. Instruct the patient to slow down breathing rate and pause longer between breaths.
C. Patient's heart rate increases more than 20 beats per minute during the treatment.
  1. Corrective action:
    a. Stop treatment immediately and notify the physician. This is most likely the result of the nebulized bronchodilator stimulating the heart.
D. The patient cannot cycle the IPPB machine off.
  1. Corrective actions:
    a. Tighten all tubing connections.
    b. Ensure there are no leaks around the mouthpiece or mask.
    c. Ensure the E-T tube or tracheostomy tube cuff is inflated adequately.
    d. If using the Bennett PR-2, check to make sure that the Bennett valve is not stuck.
    e. If using the PR-2, turn on the terminal flow control to help compensate for leaks.
    f. Check the expiratory valve function.
E. As the patient inhales, nebulization of the medication does not occur.
  1. Corrective actions:
    a. Ensure the capillary tube of the nebulizer is connected.
    b. If using the Bennett PR-2, ensure the nebulization control is turned on.
    c. Ensure the nebulizer drive line is connected.
    d. Ensure there is medication in the nebulizer.
    e. Ensure the nebulizer is positioned in an upright position.
F. During inspiration, the manometer needle stays in the negative area for the first half of the breath and then rises to the positive area during the last half.
  1. Corrective action:
    a. Increase the machine flowrate.
G. The IPPB machine repeatedly cycles on shortly after the patient has begun the expiratory phase.
  1. Corrective actions:
    a. Decrease the machine sensitivity.
    b. If using the Bird Mark 7, ensure the expiratory time for apnea control is turned off.
    c. If using the Bennett PR-2, ensure the rate control is turned off.

XI. INCENTIVE SPIROMETRY (SUSTAINED MAXIMAL INSPIRATORY THERAPY)

A. Goals of incentive spirometry
  1. **Optimize lung inflation**
     a. A sustained maximal inspiration may produce tidal volumes as high as 40 ml/kg of body weight.
     b. Ten maximal inflations should be performed every waking hour to improve distribution of ventilation, which helps prevent atelectasis and mobilize retained secretions.
  2. **Improve the cough mechanism**
  3. **Preoperative cleanup**
     a. Strengthens muscles prior to surgery
     b. Increases voluntary ventilation
     c. Improves mobilization of secretions
  4. **Reinflate areas of atelectasis**
  5. **Psychological support**
  6. **Provide early detection of pulmonary disease**
B. **Guidelines for effective incentive spirometry**
  1. Must have a motivated and cooperative patient with a **respiratory rate of less than 25/min**
  2. The patient should be able to achieve a **forced vital capacity (FVC) of greater than 15 ml/kg of body weight.**

NOTE: If the patient has an FVC of less than 15 ml/kg, IPPB therapy is indicated to improve distribution of ventilation.

C. Hazards of incentive spirometry
  1. Hyperventilation
  2. Pneumothorax (unlikely except in the COPD patient)
  3. Contaminated spirometer (except with disposables)
  4. Increased intrapleural pressure and stimulation of vagal reflex, causing decreased heart rate if the sustained maximal inspiratory pause is performed against a closed glottis (Valsalva's maneuver)
D. **Important points concerning incentive spirometry**
  1. Patient should be positioned upright in the Fowler's or semi-Fowler's position.
  2. The initial inspiratory goal should be twice the patient's tidal volume.
  3. The inspiratory time should be 5 to 15 seconds with a 2- to 3-second breath hold at end inspiration.
  4. Incentive spirometry is an alternative to IPPB if the patient can achieve an FVC of greater than 15 ml/kg of body weight.

E. Incentive spirometry devices

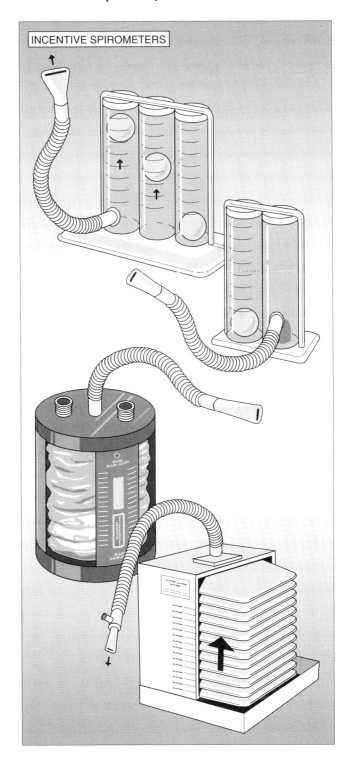

INCENTIVE SPIROMETERS

REFERENCES

Eubanks D, Bone R. *Comprehensive Respiratory Care*. 2nd ed. St. Louis: CV Mosby; 1990.

McPherson SP. *Respiratory Therapy Equipment*. 4th ed. St. Louis: CV Mosby; 1990.

Shapiro BA. *Clinical Application of Respiratory Care*. 4th ed. St. Louis: Mosby Year Book Publishers; 1990.

Scanlan C, Spearman C. *Egan's Fundamentals of Respiratory Care*. 5th ed. St. Louis: CV Mosby; 1990.

PRETEST ANSWERS

1. C

2. B

3. B

4. D

5. D

6. B

CHAPTER **7**

Cardiopulmonary Resuscitation/Manual Resuscitators

PRETEST QUESTIONS*

1. A respiratory care practitioner enters a patient's room in response to a code and finds the nurse performing CPR alone. As the first step in two-rescuer resuscitation, the practitioner should do which of the following?

A. Ask, "Are you okay?" and call the emergency medical services number.
B. Check for an airway obstruction and pupillary dilation.
C. Instruct the nurse to stop compressions and palpate for a pulse.
D. Relieve the nurse and begin one-rescuer CPR alone.

2. You enter a patient's room to give a treatment and find the patient unconscious and not breathing. What should the respiratory care practitioner do first?

A. Give two breaths.
B. Administer IPPB as ordered.
C. Perform a precordial thump.
D. Open the patient's airway.

3. While ventilating a patient with a manual resuscitator, you notice the bag is not refilling adequately. What could be the cause of this problem?

A. Malfunction of the inlet valve
B. Excessive liter flow

C. Malfunction of the exhalation valve
D. Reservoir tubing too short

4. The compression:breath ratio for one-rescuer CPR on an adult victim is which of the following?

A. 5:1
B. 15:1
C. 5:2
D. 15:2

5. A patient is being ventilated at a rate of 12/min with a Laerdal resuscitation bag. With the oxygen flow running at 8 L/min into the bag, the patient's Pa_{O_2} is 55 torr. Which of the following actions would increase the F_{IO_2} delivered to the patient?

I. Increasing the ventilation rate to 20/min
II. Increasing the oxygen flow to 15 L/min
III. Adding an oxygen reservoir to the bag

A. I only
B. I and II only
C. I and III only
D. II and III only

*See answers at the end of the chapter.

83

CHAPTER **7**

Cardiopulmonary Resuscitation/Manual Resuscitators

I. CARDIOPULMONARY RESUSCITATION (CPR) TECHNIQUES

A. **Obstructed airway (conscious adult)**
1. Determine airway obstruction by asking the victim if he/she is choking or can speak or cough.
2. Perform **abdominal thrusts** until the foreign body is expelled or the victim becomes unconscious.
3. If the victim becomes unconscious, place victim in supine position and call for help.
4. Use the tongue-jaw lift to open the mouth and perform a finger sweep with the victim's head turned to the side.
5. Open the airway using the head tilt/chin lift method.
6. Give two breaths.
7. If ventilation attempts fail (the chest does not rise or there is difficulty in expelling air into the victim), reposition the airway and ventilate again. If still no air movement, straddle the victim's thighs and perform abdominal thrusts.
8. Again perform a finger sweep and attempt ventilations.

9. Repeat sequence until the airway is cleared.
B. **Obstructed airway (unconscious adult)**
1. Determine unresponsiveness.
2. Call for help.
3. Place victim in supine position.
4. Open the airway using the head tilt/chin lift method.
5. **Determine breathlessness** by placing ear over the victim's mouth; **look, listen, and feel for air movement.**
6. Attempt to ventilate.
7. If no air movement, reposition the airway and attempt ventilation again.
8. If still no air movement, straddle the victim's thighs and perform abdominal thrusts.
9. Perform a finger sweep with the victim's head turned to the side.
10. Attempt ventilation.
11. Repeat sequence until the airway is cleared.
C. **One-rescuer CPR (adult)**
1. Determine unresponsiveness.
2. Call for help.
3. Place victim in supine position.
4. Open the airway using the head tilt/chin lift method.
5. Determine breathlessness by placing ear over the victim's mouth; look, listen, and feel for air movement.

6. Give two breaths while observing chest rise. (Allow lungs to deflate between breaths.)
7. Determine presence or absence of pulse by palpating the carotid artery.
8. If no pulse, begin chest compressions at a rate of 80 to 100 per minute (in a pattern of 15 compressions followed by 2 breaths).

NOTE: Airway, breathing, and circulation are the ABCs of CPR. Always follow this sequence.

II. ADULT, CHILD, AND INFANT CPR MODIFICATIONS

A. **Compression : ventilation ratios (one rescuer)**
   1. Adult — 15:2 at 80 to 100 compressions/min
   2. Child — 5:1 at 80 to 100 compressions/min
   3. Infant — 5:1 at >100 compressions/min
B. **Compression : ventilation ratios (two rescuers)**
   1. Adult — 5:1
   2. Child — 5:1
   3. Infant — 5:1
C. **Rescue breathing (victim with pulse)**
   1. Adult — one breath every 5 seconds
   2. Child — one breath every 4 seconds
   3. Infant — one breath every 3 seconds
D. **Compression depth**
   1. Adult — **1.5 to 2 inches** with two hands stacked, heel of one hand on lower half of the victim's sternum
   2. Child — **1 to 1.5 inches** with one hand on the lower half of the victim's sternum
   3. Infant — **0.5 to 1 inch** with two or three fingers at one finger's width below the nipple line

III. CPR — SPECIAL CONSIDERATIONS

A. **Do not** hyperextend the neck of an infant to open the airway, as this may close it off.
B. **If a manual resuscitator is not available, rescue breathing should be achieved by mouth to mouth or mouth to mask.**
C. **Never** compress the chest of a victim who has even the weakest pulse.
   1. A weak pulse probably delivers a higher cardiac output than does manual compressions.
   2. Manual compressions achieve only **25% to 35% of normal blood flow.**
D. Upon entering a room where one-rescuer CPR is

being performed, the first step to take before beginning two-rescuer CPR is to establish the presence or absence of a pulse.
E. The best indication of adequate cerebral blood flow while performing chest compressions is pupillary reaction.
F. Victims with suspected **neck injury** should have their airway opened by the **jaw thrust maneuver without head tilt.**
G. **Hazards of CPR**
   1. Rib fracture (especially in infants and the elderly; may lead to pneumothorax or lacerated liver)
   2. Fat embolism (microfractures of the ribs or sternum may cause fat to leak from bone marrow into the venous circulation)
   3. Gastric distention (from air entering the stomach during rescue breathing; air should be removed, because this interferes with lung expansion)

IV. MANUAL RESUSCITATORS

A. **Uses of manual resuscitators**
   1. Rescue breathing
   2. Hyperinflate the lungs prior to tracheal suctioning
   3. Transport patient requiring artificial ventilation
B. **The manual resuscitator**

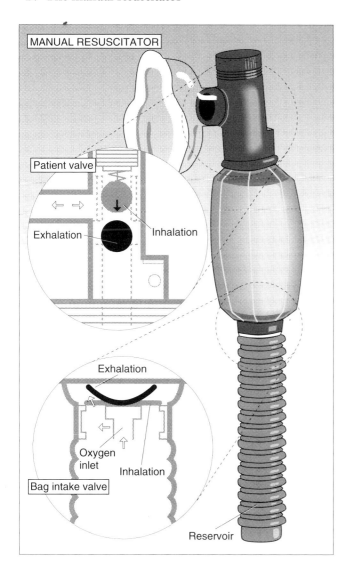

MANUAL RESUSCITATOR

Patient valve

Exhalation — Inhalation

Exhalation

Oxygen inlet — Inhalation

Bag intake valve

Reservoir

C. All resuscitators have the same basic design:
   1. A patient valve with a standard universal adaptor consisting of a 22-mm outside diameter that fits standard resuscitation masks and a 15-mm inside diameter that connects to standard endotracheal or tracheostomy tubes

2. The patient valve also houses the exhalation valve and ports that prevent the rebreathing of exhaled air.
3. The resuscitators utilize self-inflating bags with a bag intake valve.
4. A reservoir attachment should be connected to the bag intake valve so the bag reinflates with supplemental oxygen instead of room air. This will ensure that higher oxygen percentages (approaching 100%) are delivered to the patient.
5. Most resuscitator bags have pressure relief devices that open to the atmosphere at 40 cm H_2O pressure to prevent excessive pressures from being delivered to the patient's lungs.
6. **To achieve the highest delivered oxygen percentages possible, follow these criteria:**
   a. Always use a reservoir attachment if available.
   b. Use the highest flowrate that does not cause the valves to jam (10 to 15 L/min).
   c. Use the longest possible bag refill time, which means a slower ventilation rate. Allow the bag to fully refill before the next breath. A faster ventilation rate will decrease the delivered oxygen percentage.
   d. Do not use large stroke volumes (volume squeezed from the bag) if possible. Delivery of higher volumes from the bag means more room air entrained and lower oxygen percentage (not significant if a reservoir attachment is used).
D. **Hazards of using manual resuscitators**
   1. Leaks during inspiration due to improperly fitted face mask or inadequately filled E-T tube cuff
   2. Equipment malfunction due to sticking valves, missing parts, improper assembly, or dirty valve mechanisms
   3. Poor ventilation technique

E. **Mouth-to-valve mask ventilation**

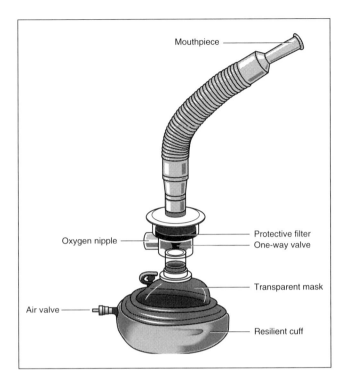

Mouthpiece

Oxygen nipple

Protective filter
One-way valve

Transparent mask

Air valve

Resilient cuff

1. This type of ventilation provides an option to mouth-to-mouth ventilation, which should not be employed in the hospital unless no other means is available.
2. Mouth-to-valve mask rescue breathing involves placing one end of the one-way valve on a mask.

The other end has a mouthpiece attached. The rescue breather may now ventilate the patient by breathing through the mouthpiece while the patient's exhaled air passes around the exhalation ports to the outside.
3. This one-way valve system for rescue breathing protects the breather from cross-contamination from the patient's exhaled air.

REFERENCES

Eubanks D, Bone R. *Comprehensive Respiratory Care.* 2nd ed. St. Louis: CV Mosby; 1990.
McPherson SP. *Respiratory Therapy Equipment.* 4th ed. St. Louis: CV Mosby; 1990.

PRETEST ANSWERS

1. C

2. D

3. A

4. D

5. D

CHAPTER **8**

Arterial Blood Gas Interpretation

NOTE: Torr and mm Hg represent the same unit and are often used interchangeably.

1. Arterial blood gas results obtained from a patient are as follows:

pH — 7.24
Pa_{CO_2} — 54 torr
HCO_3 — 25 mEq/L
Pa_{O_2} — 81 torr
B.E. — −1

You would interpret these ABG results as
A. compensated respiratory acidosis.
B. uncompensated respiratory acidosis.
C. compensated metabolic acidosis.
D. uncompensated metabolic acidosis.

2. A patient experiencing Kussmaul's respirations has the following ABG measurements:

pH — 7.18
Pa_{CO_2} — 21 torr
HCO_3 — 12 mEq/L
Pa_{O_2} — 68 torr
B.E. — −13

These ABG results would be interpreted as

A. compensated respiratory alkalosis.
B. uncompensated metabolic acidosis.
C. partially compensated metabolic acidosis.
D. compensated metabolic alkalosis.

3. Which of the following blood gas measurements determines how well a patient is ventilating?

A. pH
B. Pa_{CO_2}
C. Pa_{O_2}
D. HCO_3

4. The respiratory care practitioner has received an order to obtain ABG measurements from a patient, but an Allen's test determines that sufficient collateral circulation is not present in the right wrist. The practitioner should

A. check collateral circulation in the left wrist.
B. obtain blood from the right brachial artery.
C. obtain blood from the right radial artery.
D. obtain blood from the right femoral artery.

5. After obtaining a blood gas sample, the respiratory care practitioner should handle the sample by

A. adding heparin.
B. warming the sample.
C. placing the syringe in ice.
D. shaking the sample continuously for 15 minutes.

6. The data below are recorded for a patient with respiratory failure receiving continuous mechanical ventilation in the control mode.

FiO_2 — 0.7
Tidal volume — 500 ml
Respiratory rate — 10/min
Peak pressure — 35 cm H_2O
Pulse — 125/min
Blood pressure — 130/75

*See answers at the end of the chapter.

The patient's arterial blood gas results are as follows:
pH — 7.28
Pa_{CO_2} — 55 torr
HCO_3 — 27 mEq/L
Pa_{O_2} — 79 torr

Which of the following ventilator changes would be appropriate?
A. Increase the F_{IO_2} to 0.8.
B. Add 5 cm H_2O PEEP.
C. Decrease the respiratory rate.
D. Increase the tidal volume.

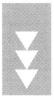

Arterial Blood Gas Interpretation

I. ARTERIAL BLOOD GAS (ABG) ANALYSIS

A. Blood gas analysis monitors the following physiologic parameters:
1. Arterial oxygenation — Pa_{O_2}
2. Alveolar ventilation — Pa_{CO_2}
3. Acid-base status — pH
4. Oxygen delivery to tissues — $P\bar{v}_{O_2}$

B. Arterial samples are used because the values reflect the patient's total cardiopulmonary status.

C. Mixed venous blood, obtained from the pulmonary artery via a Swan-Ganz catheter, is used to determine oxygen delivery to the tissues (see Chapter 9, "Ventilator Management").

D. Blood gas measurements are ordered to determine whether to change or maintain current therapy.

E. Common sites at which arterial blood is obtained are the radial, femoral, brachial, or dorsalis pedis arteries.
1. Radial artery is the most common site because of the presence of good collateral circulation and good accessibility.
2. Modified Allen's test is performed to determine collateral circulation.
   a. Patient is instructed to close hand tightly as practitioner occludes both the radial and ulnar arteries.
   b. Patient is instructed to open hand as the practitioner releases the pressure on the ulnar artery while watching for hand to return to normal color.
   c. Color should be restored in 10 to 15 seconds. If it is not, the test is considered negative, meaning collateral circulation is not present and blood **must not** be obtained from this wrist. Check collateral circulation in the other wrist.
   d. The blood sample should be placed in ice to decrease metabolic activity. This ensures a more accurate measurement.

F. Arterial blood gas sampling (via radial artery puncture)
1. Explain the procedure to the patient.
2. Perform a modified Allen test.
3. Place a folded towel under the patient's wrist to keep the wrist hyperextended.
4. Clean the puncture site with isopropyl alcohol (70%).
5. The practitioner must don gloves for this procedure.
6. A local anesthetic, such as Xylocaine (lidocaine), may be administered subcutaneously around the puncture site, especially to patients who have been punctured several times. Allow 3 to 5 minutes for the anesthetic to take effect.

7. Aspirate 0.5 ml of 1:1000 strength heparin into the syringe using a 20- or 23-gauge needle. Pull the plunger of the syringe back and forth so that the entire portion of the syringe is exposed to the heparin. The plunger should then be pushed all the way in to expel the heparin, making sure there are no air bubbles in the syringe.

NOTE: The heparin lubricates the syringe but is primarily used to prevent the blood from clotting.

8. With the needle/syringe in one hand, palpate the artery with the other. The needle should enter the skin at a 45-degree angle with the bevel pointing up. The needle should be advanced slowly until blood is pulsating into the syringe.

NOTE: Sometimes the needle will pass through the artery and only a small amount of blood enters the syringe. The needle should be slowly withdrawn until it is in the artery. If the needle needs to be redirected, it should first be withdrawn to the subcutaneous tissue.

9. After 2 to 4 ml of blood have been obtained, a sterile gauze pad should be applied with pressure over the puncture site for 3 to 5 minutes or until the bleeding has stopped.
10. Air bubbles should then be removed from the syringe since they affect the values of the blood gases. Air in the blood sample will cause elevated Pa_{O_2} levels and decreased Pa_{CO_2} levels.
11. A cap or rubber stopper should then be placed over the needle or the needle may be removed and a cap placed over the end of the syringe. This prevents air from entering the syringe.
12. The practitioner should then roll the syringe back and forth in the hands to ensure proper mixing of the blood and heparin to prevent blood clotting. The syringe is then placed in ice to slow the metabolism and keep the blood gas values accurate.
13. The practitioner should record the following information after the sample is drawn:
    a. Patient's name and room number.
    b. The F_{IO_2} the patient is on.
    c. If patient is on ventilator:
       (1) F_{IO_2}
       (2) Tidal volume
       (3) Respiratory rate
       (4) Mode of ventilation (i.e., SIMV, CMV, etc.)
       (5) PEEP
       (6) Mechanical deadspace

d. Patient's temperature—remember that a fever shifts the oxyhemoglobin curve to the right, indicating that hemoglobin more readily releases oxygen to the tissues but does not pick up the O_2 as easily. This may affect the Pa_{O_2} value, but this usually is not significant.

II. ARTERIAL OXYGENATION

A. **Partial pressure of arterial oxygen (Pa_{O_2})**
   1. The Pa_{O_2} is the portion of oxygen dissolved in the plasma of the blood or the portion that remains after the hemoglobin (Hb) molecules have been saturated.
   2. For every **1 mm Hg of Pa_{O_2}, there is 0.003 ml of dissolved oxygen.**
B. **Partial pressure of alveolar oxygen ($P_{A_{O_2}}$)**
   1. Calculated by the following formula:

$$P_{A_{O_2}} = [(P_B - 47 \text{ mm Hg}) (F_{IO_2})] - [Pa_{CO_2} \times 1.25]$$

$$P_{A_{O_2}} = (760 - 47 \text{ mm Hg}) (0.21) - 40 \text{ mm Hg} \times 1.25$$

$$P_{A_{O_2}} = (713 \times 0.21) - 50$$

$$P_{A_{O_2}} = 150 - 50 = \textbf{100 mm Hg}$$

   2. This value is often compared to Pa_{O_2} to determine P(A–a) gradient or the difference between alveolar oxygen tension and arterial oxygen tension. **Normal P(A–a) gradient for room air is 4 to 12 mm Hg.**

EXAMPLE: A patient on a 50% Venturi mask has the following ABG measurements:

pH — 7.36
Pa_{CO_2} — 45 torr
Pa_{O_2} — 94 torr

What is this patient's P(A–a) gradient? (P_B = 747 torr)

$P_{A_{O_2}}$ = [(747 – 47) (0.5)] – [45 × 1.25]
350 – 56 = 294

P(A–a) gradient = $P_{A_{O_2}}$ – Pa_{O_2}
294 – 94 = 200 torr

C. Oxyhemoglobin dissociation curve

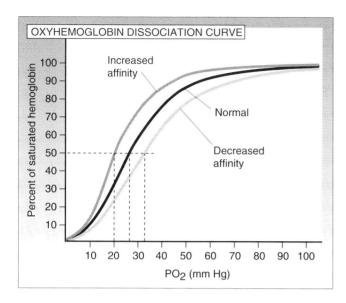

1. This curve plots the relationship between Pa_{O_2} and arterial oxygenation saturation (Sa_{O_2}) and the affinity that hemoglobin has for oxygen at various saturation levels.
2. This S-shaped curve indicates that at Pa_{O_2} levels less than 60 mm Hg, small increases in Pa_{O_2} result in fairly large increases in Sa_{O_2}. For example, 50% of the hemoglobin molecules would be carrying oxygen at a Pa_{O_2} of 26 mm Hg. As the Pa_{O_2} increases to 40 mm Hg, the Sa_{O_2} increases substantially to about 75%. As the Pa_{C_2} continues to rise to 60 mm Hg, the saturation increases to approximately 90%.
3. The flat portion of the curve indicates that at Pa_{C_2} levels above 60 mm Hg saturation rises slowly, with a Pa_{O_2} of 70 mm Hg yielding an Sa_{O_2} of 93% and Pa_{C_2} levels of between 80 to 100 mm Hg resulting in Sa_{C_2} levels of 95% to 100%.
4. Various factors affect the affinity of hemoglobin for oxygen. These factors shift the oxyhemoglobin dissociation curve to the right or the left.
5. If the curve is **shifted to the right**, it indicates that **hemoglobin's affinity for oxygen has decreased** — hemoglobin will release oxygen to the tissues more readily. **Factors that shift the curve to the right include:**
   a. Hypercapnia
   b. Acidosis
   c. Hyperthermia
   d. Increased levels of 2,3 DPG
6. If the curve is **shifted to the left**, it indicates **hemoglobin's affinity for oxygen has increased**

— hemoglobin will not release oxygen to the tissues as readily. **Factors that shift the curve to the left include:**
   a. Hypocapnia
   b. Alkalosis
   c. Hypothermia
   d. Decreased levels of 2,3 DPG
   e. Carboxyhemoglobin
7. As oxygen diffuses from the alveoli to the blood (due to pressure gradient), it enters red blood cells where it combines with hemoglobin.
8. The combination of oxygen with hemoglobin enhances the release of carbon dioxide. This is called the **Haldane effect.**
9. As RBCs travel to the tissue, they release the oxygen. The release of oxygen occurs because elevated carbon dioxide levels around tissues decrease hemoglobin's affinity for oxygen. This is known as the **Bohr effect.**
10. **Levels of hypoxemia**
    a. 60 to 79 mm Hg — mild hypoxemia
    b. 40 to 59 mm Hg — moderate hypoxemia
    c. <40 mm Hg — severe hypoxemia
11. **Normal Pa_{O_2} levels**

Age	Pa_{O_2} (torr)
<60	80 to 100
60	80
65	75
70	70
75	65
80	60

NOTE: Subtract 1 torr from 80 for each year over 60 to determine normal Pa_{O_2} by age.

12. **P 50**
    a. The P 50 represents Pa_{O_2} when the hemoglobin is 50% saturated.
    b. Normal P 50 is 26.6 torr.
    c. Used to describe hemoglobin's affinity to oxygen
       (1) Increased P 50 — decreased affinity
       (2) Decreased P 50 — increased affinity
13. **Arterial oxygen saturation (Sa_{O_2})**
    a. Refers to the quantity of oxygen carried by the hemoglobin compared with the maximum that may be carried
    b. **Normal Sa_{O_2} is 95% to 100%.**

III. CARBON DIOXIDE TRANSPORT AND ALVEOLAR VENTILATION

A. Carbon dioxide (CO_2) composes approximately 0.03% of inspired air.

B. Carbon dioxide is the by-product of cellular metabolism, the mechanism by which it enters the blood.

C. After carbon dioxide enters the blood, it takes one of two routes.

1. Five percent of the carbon dioxide dissolves in the plasma.

2. The remaining 95% enters the red blood cells.

   a. Approximately 65% of the carbon dioxide entering the RBCs is quickly converted to hydrogen and bicarbonate ions.

   b. The remaining carbon dioxide entering the RBCs combines with hemoglobin.

   c. Therefore, carbon dioxide is carried in the blood three ways:

      (1) Dissolved in the plasma

      (2) Bound to hemoglobin

      (3) As bicarbonate (HCO_3)

D. **The adequacy of ventilation is determined by the Pa_{CO_2} level.**

1. Normal Pa_{CO_2} range is 35 to 45 torr.

2. Pa_{CO_2} **<35 torr** is termed **hypocapnia** and indicates excess carbon dioxide elimination or **hyperventilation.**

3. Pa_{CO_2} **>45 torr** is termed **hypercapnia** and indicates insufficient carbon dioxide elimination or **hypoventilation.**

E. Pa_{CO_2} increases when respiratory rate or tidal volume (minute volume) decreases or dead space increases. Pa_{CO_2} decreases when respiratory rate or tidal volume increases or dead space decreases.

IV. ACID-BASE BALANCE (pH)

A. In simple terms, the pH level is determined by the amount of carbonic acid (which increases as CO_2 increases) in the blood in relation to the amount of base (HCO_3) in the blood.

1. Henderson-Hasselbalch equation states:

$$pH = pK^* + \log \frac{base}{acid}$$

2. Clinically we may state:

$$pH = pK + \log \frac{HCO_3}{P_{CO_2}^\dagger}$$

*pK represents the pH value at which the solute is 50% dissociated. It is considered the dissociation constant and = 6.1 in this equation.

†P_{CO_2} = partial pressure of carbon dioxide.

3. The important idea to remember from this equation is:

   a. **When HCO_3 (base) increases** and carbon dioxide (acid) remains unchanged, **the pH increases.**

   b. **When HCO_3 decreases** and carbon dioxide remains unchanged, the **pH decreases.**

   c. **When carbon dioxide increases** and HCO_3 remains unchanged, the **pH decreases.**

   d. **When carbon dioxide decreases** and HCO_3 remains unchanged, **the pH increases.**

In other words, HCO_3 and pH are directly proportional (if one *increases* the other *increases*), whereas CO_2 and pH are inversely proportional (if one *increases* the other *decreases*).

B. The ratio of base:acid is 20:1, which is a pH of 7.40.

C. The normal plasma pH range is 7.35 to 7.45.

1. A **pH <7.35** is termed **acidemia** and indicates a greater-than-normal hydrogen ion concentration. **Acidemia occurs as a result of:**

   a. Increased P_{CO_2} levels

   b. Decreased HCO_3 levels

2. A pH >7.45 is termed alkalemia and indicates a below-normal hydrogen ion concentration. Alkalemia occurs as a result of:

   a. Decreased P_{CO_2} levels

   b. Increased HCO_3 levels

D. **Respiratory versus metabolic components**

1. When the initial pH change is the result of a P_{CO_2} change, this is a respiratory disturbance.

   a. An **increased P_{CO_2} (>45 torr) decreases the pH (<7.35). This is termed respiratory acidosis.**

EXAMPLE: pH — 7.22
Pa_{CO_2} — 62 torr
HCO_3 — 24 mEq/L (**Normal: 22 to 26 mEq/L**)

This is **acute or uncompensated respiratory acidosis** because the **HCO_3** is still within normal limits (22 to 26 mEq/L).

   b. A decreased P_{CO_2} (**<35 torr) increases the pH (>7.45). This is termed respiratory alkalosis.**

EXAMPLE: pH — 7.56
Pa_{CO_2} — 28 torr
HCO_3 — 25 mEq/L

This is **acute or uncompensated respiratory alkalosis** because the HCO_3 is still within normal limits.

2. When the initial pH change is the result of an HCO_3 change, this is a metabolic disturbance.

a. A **decreased HCO₃ (<22 mEq/L) decreases the pH (<7.35)**. This is termed **metabolic acidosis**.

EXAMPLE: pH — 7.26
Pa_{CO_2} — 38 torr
HCO_3 — 14 mEq/L

This is **acute or uncompensated metabolic acidosis** because the Pa_{CO_2} is within normal limits.

b. An **increased HCO₃ (>26 mEq/L) increases the pH (>7.45)**. This is termed **metabolic alkalosis**.

EXAMPLE: pH — 7.56
Pa_{CO_2} — 41 torr
HCO_3 — 32 mEq/L

This is **acute or uncompensated metabolic alkalosis** because the Pa_{CO_2} is within normal limits.

E. **pH compensation**
1. The levels of HCO₃ and carbon dioxide will always change in order to keep the pH within the normal range. This is called **compensation**.
2. If the P_{CO_2} initially changes the pH, the HCO₃ will change accordingly to return the pH to normal.

EXAMPLE: (A) pH — 7.29
Pa_{CO_2} — 56 torr
HCO_3 — 30 mEq/L

(B) pH — 7.36
Pa_{CO_2} — 57 torr
HCO_3 — 34 mEq/L

The (A) example is **partially compensated respiratory acidosis**. The elevated Pa_{CO_2} caused the initial drop in pH. The HCO₃ is increasing to elevate the pH back to normal. Because the pH is approaching normal but still low, this makes it **partially compensated**. As the pH returns to normal in example (B), this is **chronic or compensated respiratory acidosis**.

EXAMPLE: (A) pH — 7.51
Pa_{CO_2} — 27 torr
HCO_3 — 18 mEq/L

(B) pH — 7.44
Pa_{CO_2} — 26 torr
HCO_3 — 13 mEq/L

The (A) example is **partially compensated respiratory**

alkalosis. The decreased Pa_{CO_2} caused the initial increase in pH. The HCO₃ is decreasing to drop the pH back to normal. Because the pH is approaching normal but still high, this makes it **partially compensated**. As the pH returns to normal in example (B), this is **chronic or compensated respiratory alkalosis**.

3. If the HCO₃ initially changes the pH, the P_{CO_2} will change accordingly to return the pH to normal.

EXAMPLE: (A) pH — 7.22
Pa_{CO_2} — 24 torr
HCO_3 — 14 mEq/L

(B) pH — 7.35
Pa_{CO_2} — 15 torr
HCO_3 — 14 mEq/L

The (A) example is **partially compensated metabolic acidosis**. The decreased HCO₃ caused the initial drop in pH. The patient is hyperventilating (decreasing P_{CO_2} levels) to elevate the pH back to normal. Because the pH is approaching normal but still low, this is **partially compensated**. As the pH returns to normal in example (B), this is **compensated metabolic acidosis**.

EXAMPLE: (A) pH — 7.51
Pa_{CO_2} — 50 torr
HCO_3 — 30 mEq/L

(B) pH — 7.45
Pa_{CO_2} — 58 torr
HCO_3 — 30 mEq/L

The (A) example is **partially compensated metabolic alkalosis**. The increased HCO₃ caused the initial increase in pH. The patient is hypoventilating (increasing P_{CO_2} levels) to drop the pH back to normal. Because the pH is approaching normal but still high, this is **partially compensated**. As the pH returns to normal in example (B), this is **compensated metabolic alkalosis**.

IMPORTANT NOTE: When interpreting a compensated blood gas measurement:

If the compensated pH is 7.35 to 7.40, the pH must be assumed to have been acidotic initially. Decide if the P_{CO_2} or HCO₃ caused the initial acidemia.

If the compensated pH is 7.40 to 7.45, the pH must be assumed to have been alkalotic initially. Decide if the P_{CO_2} or HCO₃ caused the initial alkalemia.

NOTE: **Metabolic compensation takes several hours to occur, whereas respiratory compensation may occur in minutes.**

F. **Mixed respiratory and metabolic component**
   1. If the pH increases or decreases as a result of both a P_{CO_2} change and HCO_3 change, this is called a mixed component.

EXAMPLE: pH — 7.22
          Pa_{CO_2} — 53 torr
          HCO_3 — 16 mEq/L

This is an example of **mixed respiratory and metabolic acidosis.** An elevated P_{CO_2} and decreased HCO_3 both contribute to acidemia.

V. ARTERIAL BLOOD GAS INTERPRETATION

A. **ABG normal value chart summary (Adults)**
   1. pH — 7.35 to 7.45
   2. Pa_{CO_2} — 35 to 45 mm Hg (torr)
   3. Pa_{O_2} — 80 to 100 mm Hg (torr)
   4. HCO_3 — 22 to 26 mEq/L
   5. B.E. — –2 to +2 (refers to the total base deficit or excess)
B. Normal **arterial blood gas** values for **neonates**
   1. pH — 7.30 to 7.45 (no less than 7.25 immediately after birth)
   2. Pa_{CO_2} — 35 to 45 torr
   3. Pa_{O_2} — 50 to 70 torr
   4. HCO_3 — 20 to 26 mEq/L
   5. B.E. — –5 to +5
C. Normal **capillary blood gas** values for **neonates**
   1. pH — 7.30 to 7.45
   2. Pa_{CO_2} — 35 to 50 torr
   3. Pa_{O_2} — 40 to 50 torr
   4. HCO_3 — 20 to 26 mEq/L
   5. B.E. — –5 to +5
D. Normal **arterial blood gas** values for **children**
   1. pH — 7.35 to 7.45
   2. Pa_{CO_2} — 35 to 45 torr
   3. Pa_{O_2} — 80 to 100 torr
   4. HCO_3 — 22 to 26 mEq/L
   5. B.E. — –2 to +2
E. **Basic steps to ABG interpretation**
   1. Determine the acid-base status by observing the pH.
      a. Is the pH acidotic (<7.35)?
      b. Is the pH alkalotic (>7.45)?
   2. Determine if the pH change is the result of a P_{CO_2} change or an HCO_3 change.

   3. When the cause of pH change is determined, observe for signs of compensation. If the P_{CO_2} caused the initial pH change, is the HCO_3 changing to return the pH back to normal?
   4. Determine oxygenation status by observing P_{O_2}.
F. **ABG example problems**
   1. pH — 7.26
      Pa_{CO_2} — 54 torr
      HCO_3 — 23 mEq/L
      Pa_{O_2} — 81 torr
      B.E. — –1
      a. Acid/base status: **Acidemia**
      b. Ventilatory status: **Elevated Pa_{CO_2} — hypoventilation resulting in decreased pH**
      c. Metabolic status: **Normal HCO_3 — no compensation occurring**
      d. Oxygenation status: **Normal Pa_{O_2}**
      Interpretation: **Uncompensated (acute) respiratory acidosis**
      To correct: **Institute mechanical ventilation** to increase the patient's minute volume or **increase the ventilator rate or tidal volume if already on a ventilator.**
   2. pH — 7.54
      Pa_{CO_2} — 28 torr
      HCO_3 — 24 mEq/L
      Pa_{O_2} — 94 torr
      B.E. — 0
      a. Acid/base status: **Alkalemia**
      b. Ventilatory status: **Decreased Pa_{CO_2} — hyperventilation resulting in increased pH**
      c. Metabolic status: **Normal HCO_3 — no compensation occurring**
      d. Oxygenation: **Normal Pa_{O_2}**
      Interpretation: **Uncompensated (acute) respiratory alkalosis**
      To correct: **Decrease the ventilator rate or tidal volume or add mechanical dead space.**
   3. pH — 7.40
      Pa_{CO_2} — 39 torr
      HCO_3 — 26 mEq/L
      Pa_{O_2} — 51 torr
      B.E. — +2
      a. Acid/base status: **Normal pH**
      b. Ventilation status: **Normal Pa_{CO_2}**
      c. Metabolic status: **Normal HCO_3**
      d. Oxygenation status: **Moderate hypoxemia**
      Interpretation: **Normal acid/base status with moderate hypoxemia**
      To correct: **Increase F_{IO_2}, but if patient is on 60% or more oxygen mask, place on CPAP or add PEEP on ventilator.**

4. pH — 7.36
   Pa_{CO_2} — 63 torr
   HCO_3 — 34 mEq/L
   Pa_{O_2} — 56 torr
   B.E. — +11
   a. Acid/base status: **Normal pH**
   b. Ventilatory status: **Increased Pa_{CO_2} — hypoventilation resulting in decreased pH**
   c. Metabolic status: **Elevated HCO_3 — compensating for initial acidemia**
   d. Oxygenation status: **Moderate hypoxemia**
   Interpretation: **Compensated (chronic) respiratory acidosis.** Because the compensated pH is 7.35 to 7.40, we must assume this was initially an acidemia caused by an elevated Pa_{CO_2}.
   To correct: **This is a classic example of "normal" ABG measurements for a chronic lung patient; therefore, no change in present therapy is needed.**

5. pH — 7.26
   Pa_{CO_2} — 41 torr
   HCO_3 — 14 mEq/L
   Pa_{O_2} — 90 torr
   B.E. — –8
   a. Acid/base status: **Acidemia**
   b. Ventilatory status: **Normal Pa_{CO_2}**
   c. Metabolic status: **Decreased HCO_3 resulting in decreased pH**
   d. Oxygenation status: **Normal Pa_{O_2}**
   Interpretation: **Uncompensated metabolic acidosis.** No compensation is occurring because the Pa_{CO_2} is normal.
   To correct: **Give $NaHCO_3$ (sodium bicarbonate).** No ventilator parameter changes or oxygenation modifications are necessary at this time.

6. pH — 7.19
   Pa_{CO_2} — 21 torr
   HCO_3 — 14 mEq/L
   Pa_{O_2} — 82 torr
   B.E. — –10
   a. Acid/base status: **Acidemia**
   b. Ventilatory status: **Decreased Pa_{CO_2} — hyperventilation compensating for initial acidemia**
   c. Metabolic status: **Decreased HCO_3 resulting in a decreased pH**
   d. Oxygenation status: **Normal Pa_{O_2}**
   Interpretation: **Partially compensated metabolic acidosis.** This was an initial metabolic acidosis followed by hyperventilation. By removing more carbon dioxide, the pH is returning to normal. It is not fully compensated because the pH is not

within normal limits. **This is an example of a patient with diabetic acidosis (ketoacidosis).**
To correct: **May administer $NaHCO_3$.**

G. Arterial blood gas interpretation chart

N = normal; I = increased; D = decreased

	pH	P_{CO_2}	HCO_3
Normal	N	N	N
Uncompensated (acute)			
Respiratory acidosis	D	I	N
Respiratory alkalosis	I	D	N
Metabolic acidosis	D	N	D
Metabolic alkalosis	I	N	I
Partially compensated			
Respiratory acidosis	D	I	I
Respiratory alkalosis	I	D	D
Metabolic acidosis	D	D	D
Metabolic alkalosis	I	I	I
Fully compensated (chronic)			
Respiratory acidosis	N	I	I
Respiratory alkalosis	N	D	D
Metabolic acidosis	N	D	D
Metabolic alkalosis	N	I	I
Mixed respiratory and metabolic			
Acidosis	D	I	D
Alkalosis	I	D	I

VI. BLOOD GAS ANALYZERS

A. Current blood gas analyzers have the following capabilities:
   1. Accurate measurement of pH, P_{CO_2}, and P_{O_2}
   2. Self-calibration
   3. Accurate measurement of base excess/deficit
   4. Accurate measurement of plasma bicarbonate (HCO_3)
   5. Correction for temperature
   6. Self-troubleshooting abilities
   7. Automated blood gas interpretation
B. **Blood gas electrodes**
   1. **Sanz electrode — measures pH** by quantifying the acidity and alkalinity of a solution of blood. This is accomplished by the measurement of the potential difference across a pH-sensitive glass membrane.

2. **Severinghaus electrode** — measures P_{CO_2} by causing the carbon dioxide gas to produce hydrogen ions through a chemical reaction.
3. **Clark electrode** — measures P_{O_2} as a result of a chemical reaction whereby electron flow is measured.

VII. OXYGEN SATURATION MONITORING (PULSE OXIMETRY)

A. **Use of the pulse oximeter**
1. A method by which oxyhemoglobin saturation can be measured by **spectrophotometry**
2. Light from the probe is directed through a capillary bed to be absorbed in different amounts depending on whether the hemoglobin is saturated or unsaturated. The result is displayed on the monitor as a percent of saturation.
3. The oximeter is able to find a pulsating capillary bed, which it identifies as an arterial sample.
4. The probe is noninvasive and may be attached to the finger or ear of adults and the ankle or foot of infants.
5. Pulse oximeters are quite accurate and are used to monitor the oxygenation status of a patient noninvasively. They aid in reducing F_{IO_2} levels without having to obtain blood gas measurements after each change (not used to replace ABG measurements, as pH and P_{CO_2} are not measured).

B. **Disadvantages of pulse oximeters**
1. The accuracy of pulse oximeters diminishes in the presence of low perfusion caused by:
   a. Hypotension
   b. Hypothermia
   c. Cardiac arrest
   d. Cardiopulmonary bypass
2. Accuracy diminishes in severe anemia.
3. Measurements are inaccurate when methemoglobin or carboxyhemoglobin (carbon monoxide bound to hemoglobin) is present.

VIII. TRANSCUTANEOUS MONITORING OF Pa_{CO_2} AND Pa_{O_2}

A. **Use of transcutaneous monitors**
1. Used primarily on neonates as a means of continuous, noninvasive monitoring of Pa_{CO_2} and/or Pa_{O_2}.
2. The probe is attached to the skin and heated to 42 to 44°C to increase arterialized blood flow to the dermal layer of the skin. This results in oxygen diffusion through the skin in concentrations similar to those in the arteries (Pa_{O_2} monitoring).

B. **Disadvantages of transcutaneous monitoring**
1. The patient must be hemodynamically stable.
2. The heated probe may cause burning of the skin or blisters. **To minimize this, the probe site should be changed every 3 to 4 hours!**
3. Monitors require 20 to 30 minutes to equilibrate after the initial setup or a change in probe placement.

NOTE: Normal Pa_{O_2} level in the neonate is 50 to 70 torr.

REFERENCES

Barnes TA. *Respiratory Care Practice.* St. Louis: Year Book Medical Publishers; 1988.
Eubanks D, Bone R. *Comprehensive Respiratory Care.* 2nd ed. St. Louis: CV Mosby; 1990.
Lane E. *Clinical Arterial Blood Gas Analysis.* St. Louis: CV Mosby; 1987.
Malley J. *Clinical Blood Gases: Application and Noninvasive Alternatives.* Philadelphia: WB Saunders; 1990.
McPherson SP. *Respiratory Therapy Equipment.* 4th ed. St. Louis: CV Mosby; 1990.
Shapiro BA. *Clinical Application of Blood Gases.* 4th ed. Year Book Medical Publishers; 1989.

PRETEST ANSWERS

1. B
2. C
3. B
4. A
5. C
6. D

Ventilator Management

PRETEST QUESTIONS*

1. A patient with head trauma is on the Bear 2 ventilator in the control mode. To maintain intracranial pressure within normal limits, the respiratory care practitioner should recommend which of the following?

I. Maintain Pa_{CO_2} at 25 to 30 torr.
II. Use short inspiratory times.
III. Use high peak pressures.

A. I only
B. II only
C. I and II only
D. II and III only

2. The data below pertain to an adult patient who is being mechanically ventilated.

Peak inspiratory pressure — 45 cm H_2O
Plateau pressure — 30 cm H_2O
Tidal volume — 800 ml
PEEP — 10 cm H_2O

On the basis of this information, the patient's static lung compliance is approximately which of the following?

A. 18 ml/cm H_2O
B. 23 ml/cm H_2O
C. 27 ml/cm H_2O
D. 40 ml/cm H_2O

3. The MA-1 ventilator is in the control mode and the I:E ratio alarm is sounding. Which control adjustment would correct this?

A. Increase the flowrate.
B. Increase the tidal volume.
C. Increase the respiratory rate.
D. Decrease the sensitivity.

4. The following data are collected on a ventilator patient.

V_T — 800 ml
Mode — control
F_{IO_2} — 0.60
Rate — 12/min
pH — 7.41
Pa_{CO_2} — 42 torr
Pa_{O_2} — 57 torr

The appropriate ventilator change is which of the following?

A. Increase the F_{IO_2} to 0.70.
B. Increase the tidal volume.
C. Decrease the respiratory rate.
D. Institute 5 cm H_2O of PEEP.

5. A patient is on a volume-cycled ventilator and the high pressure alarm is sounding. What is the most appropriate action to take to correct this?

A. Increase the high pressure limit.
B. Decrease the sensitivity.
C. Suction the patient's airway.
D. Increase the inspiratory flow.

*See answers at the end of the chapter.

6. A 70-kg (154-lb) patient is in respiratory failure with the following ABG measurements on a nonrebreathing mask.

pH — 7.24
Pa_{CO_2} — 58 torr
HCO_3 — 27 mEq/L
Pa_{O_2} — 62 torr

The most appropriate ventilator setting would be which of the following?

A. CPAP of 4 cm H_2O
B. SIMV — 12, V_T — 650 ml
C. SIMV — 6, V_T — 750 ml
D. SIMV — 10, V_T — 700 ml

CHAPTER 9

Ventilator Management

I. NEGATIVE- VERSUS POSITIVE-PRESSURE VENTILATORS

A. **Negative-pressure ventilators**
  1. **Iron lung** (body tank respirator)
     a. Patient is placed in an airtight cylinder up to the neck (head is exposed to ambient conditions).
     b. The underside of the cylinder has a bellows powered by an electric motor or manually operated.
     c. As the bellows descends, the pressure drops within the airtight chamber to below atmospheric pressure. This sets up a pressure gradient between the inside of the cylinder and the patient's mouth (at atmospheric pressure) and air flows into the airways.
     d. Gas flow stops as the bellows moves upward and pressures equalize. The patient exhales normally due to the elastic recoil of the lungs. (The motor moves the bellows up and down in response to a timing mechanism. Therefore the iron lung is a **time-cycled ventilator.**)
     e. The iron lung was used extensively during the polio epidemic of the 1950s. It is not commonly used to ventilate patients in current practice.
     f. Negative pressures of up to **15 cm H_2O** were commonly used to ventilate the patient.
     g. **Disadvantages of the iron lung**
        (1) Difficult patient care
        (2) Strictly a control ventilator — no means of assisting, but patient may breathe spontaneously between machine breaths.
        (3) Difficult to clean
        (4) Large and cumbersome
        (5) No means of regulating flow
        (6) "Tank shock" — pooling of abdominal blood resulting in decreased venous return
  2. **Cuirass** (chest respirator)
     a. A plastic shell that covers the chest, designed to minimize the disadvantages of the iron lung
     b. A flexible hose connects to the shell and is attached to an electric pump that creates a negative extrathoracic pressure.
     c. Because only the thorax receives negative pressure and the abdomen does not, "tank shock" was eliminated. Therefore, venous return is enhanced during inspiration.
     d. It is used to wean patients from the iron lung or for home use on paralyzed patients.
     e. **Disadvantages of the cuirass**
        (1) Noisy

(2) No means of regulating flow
(3) Difficult to maintain a tight fit
(4) Difficult patient care
   f. **Advantages of the cuirass (over the iron lung)**
     (1) Patient care is easier.
     (2) A flow-sensing device may be used to allow patient-triggered breaths.

B. **Positive-pressure ventilators**
  1. Two types of positive-pressure ventilators
    a. Preset volume ventilators (volume limited)
    b. Preset pressure ventilators (pressure limited)
  2. **Volume-limited ventilators**
    a. A preset tidal volume is delivered to the patient for each machine breath, and inspiration ends after it is delivered.
    b. The volume-limited ventilator is capable of developing an inspiratory pressure that can maintain the preset tidal volume when changes in airway resistance and compliance occur (volume constant, pressure variable).
    c. Used for mechanical ventilation of adult patients

    While routine ventilator circuit changes vary from hospital to hospital, the circuit should be changed at least once per week. Bacterial culturing of the circuits will determine whether more or less frequent circuit changes are necessary.

    The patient should be hyperoxygenated and hyperventilated prior to the changing of the ventilator circuit. In some cases, when the patient may not tolerate even the shortest time off the ventilator during the circuit change, the patient should be ventilated with a manual resuscitator by one practitioner while another changes the circuit.

  3. **Pressure-limited ventilators**
    a. A preset inspiratory pressure is delivered to the patient and inspiration ends when it is reached.
    b. The delivered tidal volume is unknown but varies with changes in airway resistance and lung compliance (volume varies, pressure constant).
    c. When lung compliance decreases, delivered tidal volume decreases. In other words, as the patient's lungs become stiffer and harder to ventilate, the delivered tidal volume decreases.
    d. The pressure control is used like the volume control. When inspiratory pressure is increased, delivered tidal volume is increased and vice versa.

    e. Used to ventilate infants and postoperative patients (wake-up) and to administer IPPB treatments. Inspiration ends on most infant ventilators when a preset time is reached. The set inspiratory pressure is reached during that time.

II. VENTILATOR CONTROLS

A. **Ventilator modes (volume ventilators)**
  1. **Control mode**
    a. Patient cannot initiate inspiration.
    b. Inspiration is initiated by a timing device. For example, at a **control rate of 10** the ventilator delivers a breath every **6 seconds** (60/10). Minute volume remains constant, as rate cannot be altered.
    c. Patient should be heavily sedated or paralyzed.
  2. **Assist mode**
    a. The patient initiates inspiration by creating a preset negative pressure that delivers a machine tidal volume.
    b. The sensitivity control determines how much negative pressure is required to initiate inspiration. It should be adjusted to –0.5 to –2 cm H_2O.
    c. The patient must initiate inspiration. There is no back-up rate should the patient become apneic. This mode is seldom used.
  3. **Assist-control mode**
    a. The patient initiates inspiration by creating a negative pressure, but if patient fails to cycle the ventilator into inspiration a back-up rate is set and a machine tidal volume breath will be delivered.
    b. This is a commonly used mode of ventilation.
    c. The patient can receive as many machine breaths as required above the set rate; therefore, the patient's minute volume is not consistent.
  4. **Intermittent mandatory ventilation (IMV)**
    a. The ventilator delivers a set number of machine breaths, but the patient is able to breathe spontaneously between machine breaths.
    b. IMV is arranged on the Bennett MA-1 ventilator by turning off the sensitivity control so that the patient cannot initiate machine breaths. A separate gas source (either a nebulizer or reservoir bag) is

attached to the inspiratory side of the circuit, providing gas for the patient to breathe spontaneously.

5. **Synchronized intermittent mandatory ventilation (SIMV)**
   a. Allows spontaneous breathing along with positive-pressure ventilator breaths. It is built into the ventilator and senses when the patient is breathing spontaneously; therefore, there is no "breath stacking."
   b. It is used both as a weaning technique and for ventilation prior to weaning but is considered mainly as a weaning mode of ventilation.
   c. The sensitivity control is left on, as the patient must create a negative pressure to allow gas flow for spontaneous breathing.
6. **Pressure support ventilation (PSV)**
   a. This is a relatively new mode of ventilation found on the new generation of ventilators that aids in the weaning process from the ventilator.
   b. It is a patient-assisted, pressure-generated, flow-cycled breath that may be augmented with SIMV or used alone.
   c. It was designed to make spontaneous breathing through the endotracheal tube during weaning more comfortable by overcoming the high resistance and increased inspiratory work caused by the E-T tube.
   d. An inspiratory pressure is set (usually 2 to 10 cm H_2O for weaning purposes). As the patient initiates inspiration, the preset pressure will be reached and held constant until a certain inspiratory flow is reached, after which the pressure is terminated.
   e. The inspiratory pressure level may be set to achieve a specific tidal volume.
   f. PSV may be used with patients who are ventilating well but are intubated to protect their airway or with patients on CPAP with oxygenation deficiencies.
7. **Continuous positive airway pressure (CPAP)**
   a. May be achieved with the use of a CPAP mask, nasal prongs, or intubation and placement on a ventilator
   b. A preset pressure is maintained in the airways as the patient breathes totally on his own. No positive-pressure breaths are delivered.
   c. Patients whose Pa_{O_2} cannot be maintained within normal limits on a **60% or more oxygen mask and who have normal or low Pa_{CO_2} levels should be placed on CPAP.** Patients with **obstructive sleep apnea benefit**

from CPAP to relieve obstruction in upper airway.
   d. Utilize **low-pressure alarm** in case of leaks.
8. **Nasal CPAP**
   a. CPAP is most commonly administered to infants with the use of nasal prongs.
   b. CPAP may also be administered with a mask, endotracheal tube, or nasopharyngeal tube.
   c. Indications for nasal CPAP
      (1) To improve oxygenation

NOTE: In order to prevent pulmonary tissue damage (ex. BPD) from high F_{IO_2} levels, CPAP should be administered. If the infant's Pa_{O_2} cannot be maintained within normal limits on a maximum of 60% oxygen hood, while Pa_{CO_2} levels remain normal or below normal, CPAP should be administered.

      (2) To increase static lung compliance
      (3) To increase functional residual capacity (FRC)
      (4) To decrease the work of breathing
      (5) To decrease intrapulmonary shunting
      (6) To decrease pulmonary vascular resistance
   d. Complications of nasal CPAP
      (1) barotrauma (pneumothorax)
      (2) decreased venous return resulting in decreased cardiac output

NOTE: These 2 complications are less likely to occur if the infant has respiratory distress syndrome (RDS) due to the reduced static lung compliance. Infants with normal lungs would be more prone to these complications.

      (3) air trapping
      (4) pressure necrosis
      (5) loss of CPAP from crying or displacement
   e. Arterial blood gases must be drawn frequently if CPAP is used to monitor Pa_{CO_2} levels. Should Pa_{CO_2} begin to rise, mechanical ventilation will be necessary.
   f. The idea of nasal CPAP on infants is based on the fact that infants are obligate nose breathers. If the baby cries, CPAP will be lost.
9. **Bilevel positive airway pressure (BiPAP)**
   a. This is a relatively new mode of intermittent mechanical ventilation that may be delivered to non-intubated patients through nasal mask or to intubated patients.
   b. BiPAP has been used to reverse chronic hypoventilation in patients with neuromus-

cular dysfunction and chest wall deformities such as kyphoscoliosis.

c. BiPAP is gaining popularity for its use in avoiding placing a patient with respiratory distress on a conventional volume-cycled ventilator.

d. BiPAP is a time-cycled, pressure-limited ventilator that allows the patient to trigger inspiration and expiration similar in nature to pressure support ventilation.

e. Inspiratory and expiratory pressures are controlled by adjustment of the inspiratory positive airway pressure (IPAP) control ranging from 2 to 25 cm H_2O and expiratory positive airway pressure (EPAP) control ranging from 2 to 20 cm H_2O.

f. The frequency control ranges from 6 to 30 cycles/min and a %IPAP control adjusts the proportion of each cycle spent at IPAP and ranges from 10 to 90%.

g. Exhaled tidal volume is also measured through the device.

B. **Tidal volume (V_T) control**

1. Determines the tidal volume delivered to the patient in milliliters or liters (variable from 50 to 2200 ml)

2. Should be set at **10 to 15 ml/kg of ideal body weight. Children: 8 to 10 ml/kg; infants: 6 to 8 ml/kg**

3. **Increasing the tidal volume increases alveolar ventilation while also increasing the minute volume. This decreases the Pa_{CO_2}.**

4. **Decreasing the tidal volume decreases alveolar ventilation while also decreasing the minute volume. This increases the Pa_{CO_2}.**

EXAMPLE: A patient breathing 10 times a minute with a tidal volume of 1000 ml has a minute volume of 10 liters. (Minute volume equals respiratory rate x tidal volume.)
If the patient begins breathing 20 times a minute with a tidal volume of 500 ml, the minute ventilation remains the same but the alveolar ventilation has decreased resulting from the decreased tidal volume.

5. On volume ventilators:

a. Increasing the tidal volume increases the inspiratory time.

b. Decreasing the tidal volume decreases the inspiratory time.

6. The preset machine tidal volume is not the actual volume reaching the patient's lungs.

a. Volume is lost in the ventilator circuit because of airway resistance from gas flow.

b. Tubing compliance may be calculated to determine how much volume is being lost in the circuit.

c. With the ventilator set on a specific tidal volume and the high pressure limit turned up completely, the machine is cycled into inspiration with the patient wye occluded. Observe the manometer pressure reading.

d. $$\text{Compliance} = \frac{\text{volume}}{\text{pressure}}$$

EXAMPLE: Set V_T — 200 ml (0.2 L)
Peak pressure reached — 40 cm H_2O

$$C = \frac{200 \text{ ml}}{40 \text{ cm } H_2O} = 5 \text{ ml/cm } H_2O$$

This means that once the patient is placed on the ventilator, 5 ml of the dialed-in volume will be lost in the tubing for every cm H_2O registering on the manometer.

EXAMPLE: Tubing compliance — 5 ml/cm H_2O
V_T — 800 ml
Peak inspiratory pressure — 20 cm H_2O

Lost volume = tubing compliance x peak inspiratory pressure

$$5 \text{ ml/cm } H_2O \text{ x } 20 \text{ cm } H_2O = \textbf{100 ml}$$

Dialed-in tidal volume = 800 ml – 100 ml (lost volume) = **700 ml**

e. Lost volume is affected by the water level in the humidifier. Lower water levels allow more compressed volume into the walls of the humidifier, resulting in more lost volume and less volume delivered to the patient.

f. More volume will be lost in the patient's conducting airways (trachea, bronchi, etc.) owing to resistance to gas flow. This part of the patient's airway is called the **anatomic dead space.** It is the part of the airway where no gas exchange occurs and is often called "wasted air."

NOTE: **Anatomic dead space is equal to 1 ml/lb (2.2 lb = 1 kg) of the patient's ideal body weight but is reduced by 50% in the intubated patient. Thus, anatomic dead space equals 1 ml/kg (2.2 lb = 1 kg).**

EXAMPLE: **A 75-kg (165-lb) patient has an anatomic dead space of approximately 75 ml.** This means that 75 ml of the patient's tidal volume does not reach the alveoli to take part in gas exchange. This figure may be subtracted from the ventilator tidal volume setting to obtain a corrected tidal volume.

NOTE: When using 10 to 15 ml/kg of body weight as the formula for selecting ventilator tidal volume, the lost volume is taken into account and this is usually an adequate tidal volume.

7. Exhaled tidal volume is measured with a bellows spirometer (MA-1) or by a digital readout. It is most accurately measured with a respirometer placed between the E-T tube and ventilator wye or at the exhalation valve. **The tidal volume delivered by the ventilator should be measured at the ventilator outlet.**
8. Volume may be lost from other causes.
   a. Loose humidifier jar or tubing connections — registers a low exhaled tidal volume reading on spirometer
   b. Leak around E-T tube cuff — low exhaled tidal volume reading
9. If the bellows spirometer on the MA-1 ventilator rises during inspiration (it should drop), the most likely cause is a hole in the exhalation diaphragm or a disconnected exhalation drive line.
10. If the bellows spirometer fails to empty during inspiration, check dump valve or reconnect dump valve tubing.

C. Respiratory rate control
   1. **Normal initial setup is 8 to 12 breaths/min.**
   2. **Adjusting the rate control alters the expiratory time, thereby altering the I:E ratio.**
      a. Increasing rate decreases expiratory time.
      b. Decreasing rate increases expiratory time.
   3. **Adjusting the rate alters the minute ventilation.**
      a. Increasing rate increases minute ventilation.
      b. Decreasing rate decreases minute ventilation.
   4. **Adjusting the rate affects the Pa_{CO_2} level.**
      a. Increasing rate decreases Pa_{CO_2}.
      b. Decreasing rate increases Pa_{CO_2}.

NOTE: Adjusting the rate to alter the patient's Pa_{CO_2} level is more beneficial for patients on controlled ventilation or SIMV/IMV. On assist/control the patient may obtain as many machine breaths as needed regardless of the rate setting.

   5. Adjustable on most ventilators from 0.5 to 60 breaths/min

D. Flowrate control
   1. Normal setting — 40 to 60 L/min
   2. Adjusting the flowrate alters the inspiratory time, thereby altering the I:E ratio.
      a. Increasing flowrate decreases inspiratory time.
      b. Decreasing flowrate increases inspiratory time.
   3. Adjustable on most ventilators from 20 to 120 L/min

E. **I:E ratio**
   1. A comparison of the inspiratory time to the expiratory time
   2. **Normal I:E ratio for the adult is 1:2. This means that expiration time should be twice as long as inspiration.**
   3. Normal I:E ratio for the infant is 1:1.
   4. The I:E ratio is established by the use of **three** ventilator controls on the volume ventilator.
      a. **Volume control**
         (1) Increasing volume increases inspiratory time.
         (2) Decreasing volume decreases inspiratory time.
      b. **Flowrate control**
         (1) Increasing flowrate decreases inspiratory time.
         (2) Decreasing flowrate increases inspiratory time.
      c. **Respiratory rate control**
         (1) Increasing rate decreases expiratory time.
         (2) Decreasing rate increases expiratory time.
   5. I:E ratio is calculated by the following formula:

$$\frac{\text{inspiratory flowrate (L/min)}}{\text{minute ventilation (L/min)}} - 1 \text{ (for inspiration)}$$

EXAMPLE: V_T — 800 ml (0.8 L)
  Rate — 12/min
  Flow — 40 L/min

$$\text{I:E ratio} = \frac{40 \text{ L/min}}{9.6 \text{ L/min}} = 4.2 - 1 = \mathbf{1{:}3.2}$$
$$(0.8 \text{ L} \times 12)$$

   6. Inspiratory time should not generally exceed expiratory time. This is termed **an inverse I:E ratio.** It may greatly compromise venous blood return to the heart.
      a. If I:E ratio alarm is sounding on the ventilator, three controls may be altered to correct it:
         (1) Rate — decrease to lengthen expiratory time
         (2) Volume — decrease to shorten inspiratory time

NOTE: Because altering one of these two controls would change the minute volume, they normally are not changed to correct inverse I:E ratio.

        (3) Flow — increase to shorten inspiratory time; **most common adjustment to correct for an inverse I:E ratio**

F. Oxygen percentage control
1. Adjustable from 21% to 100% to maintain normal Pa_{O_2} levels
2. Oxygen percentage should be increased to a maximum of 60% to maintain normal Pa_{O_2} levels. When 60% is reached, PEEP should be added or increased.
3. Oxygen should first be reduced to a level of 60% before decreasing PEEP levels in hyperoxygenated patients.

G. Sensitivity control
1. Determines the amount of patient effort required to cycle the ventilator into inspiration
2. Should be set so the patient will pull a **negative 0.5 to 2 cm H_2O pressure**
3. If the ventilator self-cycles, the sensitivity is too high. Decrease the sensitivity.
4. **If it takes more than –2 cm H_2O pressure to cycle the ventilator into inspiration, increase the sensitivity.**
5. In the control mode of ventilation, the sensitivity is turned off, prohibiting the patient from triggering a machine breath.
6. The sensitivity is also turned off on the MA-1 ventilator when using an external gas source for the IMV mode.
7. On the MA-1, when PEEP is added or increased the sensitivity must be increased accordingly and decreased if PEEP is decreased to maintain the patient effort needed to trigger a machine breath at –2 cm H_2O.

H. **Low-pressure alarm**
1. Should be set 5 to 10 cm H_2O pressure below peak inspiratory pressure
2. This audible and visual alarm will be activated by leaks in the ventilator circuit as well as by disconnection of the patient from the ventilator.
3. This is a very important monitoring alarm for patients who are paralyzed or those on CPAP.

I. **High-pressure limit**
1. Should be set 5 to 15 cm H_2O above normal peak inspiratory pressure.
2. High-pressure limit alarm may be activated by:
   a. Increasing airway resistance
   b. Decreasing lung compliance
   c. Water in the ventilator tubing
   d. Kink in the ventilator tubing

   e. Patient coughing
   f. Bronchospasm
   g. Secretions in the airway

J. Sigh controls
1. Sigh rate should be set at 6 to 12 sighs per hour.
2. Sigh volume should be set at 1.5 to 2 times the tidal volume.
3. Sighs aid in preventing atelectasis.
4. Usually not functional in the SIMV mode

NOTE: When using 10 to 15 mL/kg tidal volumes, sighs may not be necessary. They also may lead to a higher incidence of barotrauma and cardiac side effects resulting from the larger volume and pressure and longer inspiratory time.

K. **Inflation hold**
1. Adjustable from 0 to 2 seconds
2. Mechanism keeps the exhalation valve closed, causing the ventilator tidal volume to be held in the lungs for a preset time.
3. Used to improve oxygenation by reducing atelectasis and shunting and increasing the diffusion of gases
4. Using the inspiratory hold or plateau causes an increased intrathoracic pressure.
5. Used to obtain a plateau pressure to calculate static lung compliance.

L. **Positive end-expiratory pressure (PEEP)**
1. Used to maintain positive pressure in the airway following a ventilator breath
2. **Indications for PEEP**
   a. Atelectasis
   b. Hypoxemia on oxygen percentage 60% or higher
   c. Decreased functional residual capacity (FRC)
   d. To lower oxygen percentage to safe levels (<60%)
   e. Decreased lung compliance
   f. Pulmonary edema
3. **Hazards of PEEP**
   a. Barotrauma
   b. Decreased venous return
   c. Decreased cardiac output
   d. Decreased urinary output
4. Excessive PEEP levels may lead to decreases in Pa_{O_2} and lung compliance by overdistending already-open alveoli and shunting blood to collapsed alveoli.
5. If PEEP causes a decreased cardiac output, this will be evidenced by a drop in blood pressure and $P\bar{v}_{O_2}$ values.
6. **Optimal PEEP — the level of PEEP that**

improves lung compliance without decreasing the cardiac output.

7. A mixed venous P_{O_2} ($P\overline{v}_{O_2}$) may be obtained from the pulmonary artery via the Swan-Ganz catheter.

   a. Normal $P\overline{v}_{O_2}$ is 35 to 45 mm Hg.

   b. A $P\overline{v}_{O_2}$ of less than 35 mm Hg indicates a possible decrease in cardiac output. If the $P\overline{v}_{O_2}$ drops after initiation of PEEP, this is a good indicator of reduced venous return and cardiac output caused by the PEEP.

   c. The $P\overline{v}_{O_2}$ value represents the adequacy of tissue oxygenation.

   d. Use the PEEP level that provides the best lung compliance and $P\overline{v}_{O_2}$ value.

8. PEEP pressure curves compared to other curves

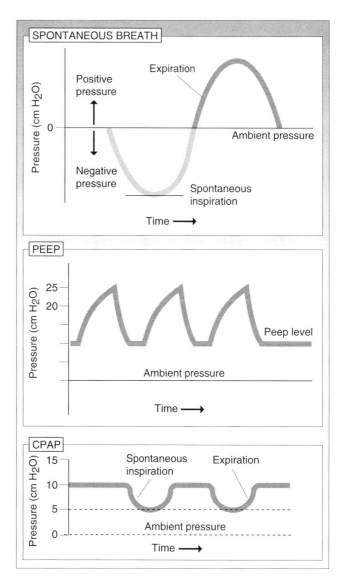

III. INDICATIONS FOR MECHANICAL VENTILATION

A. **Apnea**

B. **Acute ventilatory failure**

   1. Pa_{O_2} of greater than 50 mm Hg indicates ventilatory failure and a need for mechanical assistance.

   2. To determine ventilatory failure in a COPD patient who chronically retains carbon dioxide, observe a pH below normal to determine the need for ventilator assistance.

C. **Impending acute ventilatory failure**

   1. Sometimes normal ABG values can be deceiving. A patient may have normal ABG measurements

but be breathing 30 to 40 times per minute to achieve a normal P_{CO_2} level. Such a patient is likely to tire quickly, with an elevated Pa_{CO_2} level resulting in ventilatory failure.

2. A patient with a neuromuscular disease such as <u>Guillain-Barré syndrome must be monitored closely for lung muscle involvement.</u> **Measurement of the patient's negative inspiratory force will best determine the lung status.**

D. Oxygenation
1. Patient may be ventilating adequately but oxygenating poorly.
2. Mechanical ventilation is indicated if oxygen deficiency is directly related to an abnormal ventilatory pattern or an increased work of breathing.
3. A patient on an oxygen mask of **60% or higher** <u>ventilating well (normal or low Pa_{CO_2}) but not oxygenating adequately (low Pa_{O_2}) is probably exhibiting a large intrapulmonary shunt. This may be corrected by the use of CPAP. Mechanical ventilation may not be necessary initially.</u>

IV. COMMON CRITERIA FOR INITIATION OF MECHANICAL VENTILATION

A. Vital capacity of less than 15 ml/kg (normal is 65 to 75 ml/kg)
B. Alveolar-arterial [P(A–a)] gradient of greater than 350 mm Hg on 100% oxygen (normal is 25 to 65 mm Hg)
1. When the Pa_{O_2} is low and the P(A–a) gradient is normal for ambient conditions and the patient's age, hypoxemia is most likely the result of hypoventilation.
2. When the Pa_{O_2} is low and the P(A–a) gradient is high, hypoxemia is most likely the result of either a ventilation/perfusion mismatch, diffusion defect, or shunting. In this type of situation the patient may be hyperventilating to compensate for the hypoxemia.
C. V_D/V_T ratio greater than 60% (normal is 25% to 35%)

$$\frac{V_D}{V_T} = \frac{Pa_{CO_2} - P\bar{E}_{CO_2}}{Pa_{CO_2}}$$

D. Negative inspiratory force (NIF) less than –20 cm H_2O (normal is –50 to –100 cm H_2O)

NOTE: Negative inspiratory force is also referred to as maximal inspiratory pressure (MIP).

E. Peak expiratory pressure (PEP) less than 40 cm H_2O (normal is 100 cm H_2O)

NOTE: A NIF less than –20 cm H_2O or a PEP less than 40 cm H_2O indicates the patient cannot generate an adequate cough to maintain secretion clearance.

F. Respiratory rate greater than 35/min (normal is 10 to 20/min)

V. GOALS OF MECHANICAL VENTILATION

A. Increased minute ventilation
B. Decreased work of breathing
C. Increased alveolar ventilation
D. Maintain ABG values within normal range
E. Improved distribution of inspired gases — it has been shown that positive-pressure breathing on 21% oxygen increases Pa_{O_2} slightly.

VI. COMPLICATIONS OF MECHANICAL VENTILATION

A. **Barotrauma**
1. Pneumothorax — may be evident due to **subcutaneous emphysema** (air in the subcutaneous tissues)
2. Pneumomediastinum
3. Pneumopericardium
B. **Pulmonary infection**
1. Debilitated patients have lower resistance
2. Contaminated equipment
3. Improper airway care (tracheostomy care, suctioning, etc.)
4. Retained secretions due to E-T tube and poor cough
5. Ciliary dysfunction due to E-T tube

NOTE: The most cost-effective method of preventing cross-contamination of patients and equipment is proper hand-washing technique.

C. Atelectasis
1. Use a minimum tidal volume of 10 ml/kg of body weight to prevent atelectasis.
2. Instituting a sigh breath periodically reduces the potential of atelectasis.
3. Some believe that sighs are not necessary if V_T of 10 to 15 ml/kg of ideal body weight is used.

D. **Pulmonary oxygen toxicity**
 1. Also known as adult respiratory distress syndrome (ARDS)
 2. Caused by high oxygen concentrations for prolonged periods of time
 3. Characterized by:
   a. Impaired surfactant production
   b. Capillary congestion
   c. Edema
   d. Fibrosis
   e. Thickening of alveolar membranes
   f. Decreased lung compliance resulting in high peak pressures required to ventilate the patient

NOTE: See Chapter 10, "Lung Disorders," for more information.

E. **Tracheal damage** — usually at the cuff site
F. **Decreased venous blood return to the heart**
 1. Results from transfer of positive airway pressures to the large veins returning blood to the heart. This results in decreased pulmonary blood flow, decreased cardiac output, and decreased blood pressure.
G. **Decreased urinary output**
 1. Results from decreased renal blood flow (due to decreased cardiac output)
 2. Also results from an increased production of antidiuretic hormone (ADH)
   a. ADH production is increased due to baroreceptors in the atria of the heart that sense the decreased venous return.
   b. These receptors send a message to the hypothalamus, which stimulates the pituitary gland to secrete more ADH, thereby inhibiting urine excretion.
H. **Lack of nutrition**
 1. Malnutrition may lead to:
   a. Difficulty weaning from the ventilator due to weakened respiratory muscles
   b. Reduced response to hypoxia and hypercapnia
   c. Impaired wound healing
   d. Decreased surfactant production
   e. Infection
   f. Pulmonary edema due to decreased serum albumin levels
 2. Because oral feeding is not possible, nasogastric feedings should be implemented. Other feeding methods include the intravenous route or enteral feedings through a catheter in the stomach.
 3. High-protein, high-carbohydrate diets are recommended.

VII. DEAD SPACE

A. Dead space is that portion of the tidal volume that does not take part in gas exchange.
B. Types of dead space
 1. **Anatomic dead space** — consists of the conducting airways from the nose and mouth to the terminal bronchioles and air that does not reach the alveolar epithelium where gas exchange occurs.
   a. Anatomic dead space — 1 ml/lb body weight
   b. **A tracheostomy decreases the anatomic dead space by 50%** due to bypassing the upper airway.
 2. **Alveolar dead space**
   a. Air reaching the alveoli but not taking part in gas exchange
   b. Results from lack of perfusion to air-filled alveoli
   c. May result from hyperinflated alveoli in which blood is not able to utilize all the air
 3. **Physiologic dead space**
   a. The sum of anatomic and alveolar dead space
   b. The most accurate measurement of dead space
 4. **Determining alveolar ventilation**
   $(V_T - \text{anatomic } V_D) \times \text{respiratory rate}$

NOTE: Anatomic deadspace is equal to 1 ml/lb of ideal body weight.

EXAMPLE: A 165-lb (75-kg) male patient is breathing 12 times per minute with an average tidal volume of 500 ml. Calculate this patient's alveolar ventilation.

$$(500 \text{ ml} - 165 \text{ ml}) \times 12 =$$
$$335 \text{ m} \times 12 = 4020 \text{ ml or } 4.02 \text{ L}$$

 5. **Mechanical dead space**
   a. Ventilator circuits have a certain amount of dead space that ranges from 75 to 150 ml.
   b. Because anatomic dead space decreases when a patient is intubated or has undergone tracheotomy, the dead space created by the circuit is balanced out.
   c. Additional mechanical dead space may be added to the ventilator circuit **between the ventilator wye and the E-T tube adaptor to increase Pa$_{CO_2}$ levels.**
    (1) For every 100 ml of dead space added, the Pa$_{CO_2}$ increases approximately 5 mm Hg.
    (2) Mechanical dead space should be added

to the circuits of patients on control or assist-control only. **Never add dead space if the patient is on SIMV/IMV or CPAP.**

VIII. LUNG COMPLIANCE

A. Compliance is defined as the change in volume that corresponds to the change in pressure accompanying the volume change.

$$C = \frac{V}{P}$$

1. Lung compliance is the ease with which the lung expands.
2. The higher the compliance, the easier it is to ventilate the lung.
3. The lower the compliance, the stiffer the lung is and the harder it is to ventilate.
4. **Normal total lung compliance** (sum of lung tissue and thoracic cage) is **0.1 L/cm H_2O.**

B. **Calculation of lung compliance**
   1. **Dynamic compliance**
      a. $\dfrac{V_T}{PIP - PEEP}$

EXAMPLE: Given the following data, calculate the patient's dynamic lung compliance.

$$V_T — 600 \text{ ml}$$
$$PIP — 35 \text{ cm } H_2O$$
$$PEEP — 5 \text{ cm } H_2O$$

Dynamic compliance = $\dfrac{600 \text{ ml}}{\underset{(35 - 5)}{30 \text{ cm } H_2O}}$ = **20 ml/cm H_2O**

   b. Dynamic compliance is measured as air is flowing through the circuit and airways; therefore, it is actually a measurement of airway resistance.
   c. Dynamic compliance will change with changes in airway resistance caused by:
      (1) Water in the ventilator tubing
      (2) Bronchospasm
      (3) Secretions
      (4) Mucosal edema
   d. Dynamic compliance is not an accurate measure of lung compliancy.
   2. **Static compliance**
      a. A more accurate measurement of lung compliance or how easily the lung is ex-

panded, as it is measured with no air flowing through the circuit and airways (static conditions)
   b. Air flow may be stopped with the volume remaining in the lungs by adjusting a 1- to 2-second inspiratory hold or pinching off the expiratory drive line after inspiration has begun.
   c. After the flow has stopped, a **plateau pressure** will occur after peak pressure has been reached.
   d. Static compliance is calculated as follows:

$$\frac{V_T}{\text{Plateau pressure} - PEEP}$$

EXAMPLE: V_T — 800 ml
Plateau pressure — 25 cm H_2O
PEEP — 5 cm H_2O
Peak pressure — 45 cm H_2O

Calculate the static lung compliance.

$$\frac{800 \text{ ml}}{\underset{(25 - 5)}{20 \text{ cm } H_2O}} = \textbf{40 ml/cm } H_2O$$

NOTE: The tidal volume value used in calculating compliance may be the dialed-in volume, but most accurately would be the exhaled volume measured at the patient's ventilator wye connector with a respirometer.

C. **Important points concerning lung compliance**
   1. Increasing plateau pressures indicate the lung compliance is decreasing or the lungs are harder to ventilate.
   2. If the peak pressures are increasing but the plateau pressure remains the same, then lung compliance is not decreasing; instead, an increased airway resistance is occurring (bronchospasm, secretions, etc.).

EXAMPLE:

Time	Peak Pressure	Plateau Pressure
6 AM	28 cm H_2O	10 cm H_2O
7 AM	34 cm H_2O	10 cm H_2O
8 AM	42 cm H_2O	10 cm H_2O

In this example, the peak pressures are increasing while

the plateau pressures are remaining stable. This indicates an increase in airway resistance and not a decreasing lung compliance.

EXAMPLE:

Time	Peak Pressure	Plateau Pressure
1 PM	34 cm H_2O	16 cm H_2O
2 PM	40 cm H_2O	23 cm H_2O
3 PM	44 cm H_2O	25 cm H_2O

In this example, the plateau pressures are increasing along with the peak pressures. **This indicates a decreasing lung compliance.**

   3. Decreasing static lung compliance results from:
     a. Pneumonia
     b. Pulmonary edema
     c. Consolidation
     d. Atelectasis
     e. Air trapping
     f. Pleural effusion
     g. Pneumothorax
     h. ARDS
   4. Normal static lung compliance of the ventilated patient is 60 to 70 ml/cm H_2O.

IX. VENTILATION OF THE HEAD TRAUMA PATIENT

A. Higher-than-normal flowrates should be used to make inspiratory time shorter, lessening the time of positive pressure in the airways. The longer the time of positive pressure in the airways, the more impedance of blood flow from the head, which increases intracranial pressure (ICP).
B. Maintain the Pa_{CO_2} **at 25 to 30 mm Hg,** as this reduces ICP by vasoconstriction of cerebral vessels. **ICP should be maintained below 15 mm Hg (normal ICP is <10 mm Hg).**
C. If the ICP begins to increase, the patient should be hyperventilated (preferably with a resuscitation bag) to reduce the cerebral blood flow, thus lowering ICP.
D. Caution must be exercised when suctioning, as this tends to increase ICP due to hypoxemia.

X. WEANING FROM MECHANICAL VENTILATION

A. **Criteria for weaning**
   1. Tidal volume equal to three times the body weight in kg
   2. Vital capacity >15 ml/kg or twice the tidal volume
   3. NIF > –20 cm H_2O
   4. $V_D:V_T$ ratio of <0.60
   5. P(A–a) gradient <350 mm Hg on 100% oxygen
   6. Respiratory rate of less than 25/min
   7. Patient should be alert and able to follow commands.
   8. Patient should be off any medications that may hinder spontaneous ventilation.
   9. Life-threatening situations such as shock or hypotension should not be present.
  10. Anemia, fever, or electrolyte imbalances should not be present.
B. **Weaning techniques**
   1. Using SIMV/IMV to decrease the number of mechanical ventilator breaths while allowing for more spontaneous breathing
     a. Patient should be on 40% oxygen or less prior to extubation.
     b. Patient should be on SIMV/IMV rate of four or less before removal from the ventilator.
     c. Postoperative patients may be weaned as they awake. If they have normal blood gas values and are beginning to arouse, the SIMV/IMV rate may be decreased.
   2. **Time on/time off method**
     a. Patient is taken off the ventilator periodically and placed on flow-by for a specific length of time, then placed back on the ventilator.
     b. The time off the ventilator is gradually increased until the patient is spending more time off the ventilator than on.
     c. Patient is often returned to the ventilator while asleep.
     d. Patient must be monitored closely (blood pressure, tidal volume, heart rate, respiratory rate, and oxygen saturation/ABG measurements)
     e. The oxygen percentage is often increased by 10% while on flow-by.

XI. PRACTICE VENTILATOR PROBLEMS

A. A 75-kg male patient has been intubated and the physician wants your recommendation for ventilator settings. Which settings should be recommended?

    A. V_T — 700 ml, rate — 14
    B. V_T — 1100 ml, rate — 8
    C. V_T — 850 ml, rate — 6
    D. V_T — 700 ml, rate — 12

Answer: B. The tidal volume is in the 10- to 15-ml/kg range and the rate falls between 8 to 12 breaths/min. **Remember, an adequate initial rate setting is 8 to 12 breaths/min.**

B. A spontaneously breathing patient in the ICU has pneumonia and is set up on a 60% oxygen mask. ABG results are:
pH — 7.51
Pa_{CO_2} — 29 torr
Pa_{O_2} — 48 torr
What is the most appropriate recommendation?

    A. Increase oxygen to 80%.
    B. Place on controlled mechanical ventilation.
    C. Place on CPAP.
    D. Deliver aerosolized antibiotics.

Answer: C. Patient is ventilating well but is oxygenating poorly on 60% oxygen. Sixty percent is the high limit of oxygen, so place on CPAP to improve oxygenation.

C. A 38-year-old, 70-kg (154-lb) male is being mechanically ventilated after abdominal surgery. Ventilator settings are as follows:
Mode — SIMV
FIO_2 — 0.40
Rate — 12
V_T — 800 ml
ABG measurements reveal:
pH — 7.45
Pa_{CO_2} — 35 torr
Pa_{O_2} — 58 torr
What is the most appropriate recommendation?

    A. Increase rate to 15.
    B. Increase V_T to 950 ml.
    C. Add mechanical dead space.
    D. Increase FIO_2 to 0.5.

Answer: D. The only problem with this patient is moderate hypoxemia.

D. A patient in the control mode of ventilation is on the following settings:
V_T — 600 ml
Rate — 10
FIO_2 — 0.45
ABG results are as follows:
pH — 7.28
Pa_{CO_2} — 59 torr
HCO_3 — 26 mEq/L
Pa_{O_2} — 79 torr
What would be the most appropriate ventilator change to make?

    A. Increase V_T to 700 ml.
    B. Add 5 cm H_2O PEEP.
    C. Place on SIMV of 8.
    D. Add 100 ml of mechanical dead space.

Answer: A. This patient is not ventilating adequately (increased Pa_{CO_2}). To decrease the Pa_{CO_2} the minute volume must be increased. This is done by increasing either the rate or tidal volume.

E. A 65-kg (143-lb) female patient is on the MA-1 ventilator on the following settings:
Mode — control
V_T — 1000 ml
Rate — 12
FIO_2 — 0.40
ABG results reveal:
pH — 7.54
Pa_{CO_2} — 28 torr
Pa_{O_2} — 104 torr
What is the appropriate ventilator change?

    A. Decrease FIO_2 to 0.30.
    B. Increase V_T to 1200 ml.
    C. Decrease rate to 4.
    D. Decrease V_T to 800 ml.

Answer: D. The tidal volume setting is more than 15 ml/kg; therefore, the patient is being hyperventilated. The FIO_2 need not be decreased, as the Pa_{O_2} will decrease as the volume is reduced.

XII. VENTILATOR FLOW WAVE CAPABILITIES

A. Square wave (constant flow)

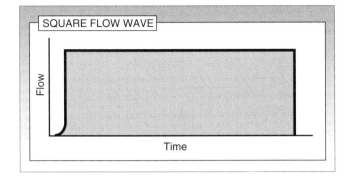

1. With this flow pattern, the flow remains constant throughout inspiration.
2. Changes in airway resistance and compliance will not change the flow pattern under normal circumstances.
3. This type of flow pattern is beneficial to patients with increased respiratory rates.

B. Sine wave

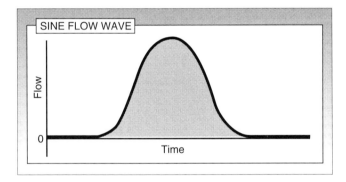

1. Flow gradually accelerates from the beginning of inspiration, then decelerates toward the end of inspiration.
2. This flow pattern benefits patients with increased airway resistance by decreasing airway turbulence.

C. Decelerating flow wave

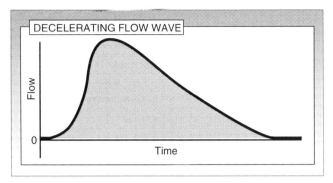

1. Initial flow is high and begins decelerating as inspiration continues.
2. Flow will never decrease more than 50% to 55% of initial flow.
3. Benefits patients with low compliance, as this pattern allows ventilation to occur at a decreased pressure.

D. Accelerating flow wave

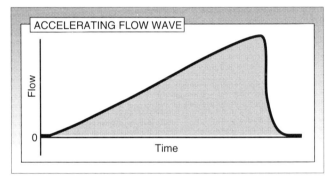

1. Flow is initially slow and accelerates to a peak flow by the end of inspiration.
2. This pattern creates less turbulence of flow at the beginning of inspiration; therefore, more volume may be delivered through narrowed or obstructed airways.

XIII. SUMMARY OF VENTILATOR ADJUSTMENTS ACCORDING TO ARTERIAL BLOOD GAS RESULTS

ABG Abnormality	Ventilator Adjustment
Decreased pH Increased Pa_{CO_2} Decreased or normal Pa_{O_2}	Increase tidal volume (maintain 10 to 15 ml/kg) Increase rate
Increased pH Decreased Pa_{CO_2}	Decrease tidal volume Decrease rate Add mechanical dead space
Normal pH Increased Pa_{CO_2} Pa_{O_2} 50 to 60 torr	No adjustment needed, as this is a COPD patient May place on SIMV
Normal pH Normal Pa_{CO_2} Decreased Pa_{O_2}	Increase F_{IO_2} if <0.60 Add or increase PEEP if F_{IO_2} is 0.60 or greater
Normal pH Normal Pa_{CO_2} Increased Pa_{O_2}	Decrease F_{IO_2} if greater than 0.60 Decrease PEEP if F_{IO_2} is less than 0.60
Decreased pH Normal Pa_{CO_2} Decreased HCO_3	No ventilator changes are necessary Administer HCO_3

REFERENCES

Eubanks D, Bone R. *Comprehensive Respiratory Care.* 2nd ed. St. Louis: CV Mosby; 1990.

Dupuis YG. *Ventilators: Theory and Clinical Application.* St. Louis: CV Mosby; 1986.

McPherson SP. *Respiratory Therapy Equipment.* 4th ed. St. Louis: CV Mosby; 1990.

Pilbeam SP. *Mechanical Ventilation: Physiological and Clinical Applications.* St. Louis: CV Mosby; 1992.

Scanlan C, Spearman C. *Egan's Fundamentals of Respiratory Care.* 5th ed. St. Louis: CV Mosby; 1990.

PRETEST ANSWERS

1. C
2. D
3. A
4. D
5. C
6. D

Lung Disorders

PRETEST QUESTIONS*

1. What would be the most appropriate recommendation for a patient suffering from obstructive sleep apnea?

A. Sleep in the supine position.
B. Sleep in Trendelenburg's position.
C. Sleep with nonrebreathing mask.
D. Use nasal CPAP while sleeping.

2. Which of these refers to a localized collection of pus in the pleural space?

A. Pulmonary edema
B. Lung abscess
C. Cyst
D. Empyema

3. A 14-year-old boy with a past history of seasonal wheezing enters the emergency room in moderate distress and complains of shortness of breath for the past hour. This patient's blood gases would most likely reveal

A. respiratory acidosis.
B. respiratory alkalosis.
C. metabolic acidosis.
D. metabolic alkalosis.

4. Digital clubbing is the result of

A. chronic hypercapnia.
B. chronic hypoxemia.
C. acute hypercapnia.
D. acute hypoxemia.

5. Sputum culture and sensitivity would be most helpful for evaluating which of the following clinical conditions?

A. Pneumonitis
B. Pleural effusion
C. Pneumothorax
D. Pulmonary edema

6. When inspecting the chest of a patient with emphysema, the respiratory care practitioner would most likely find which of the following?

A. Asymmetrical chest excursion
B. Obesity
C. Barrel chest
D. Paradoxical chest movement

*See answers at the end of the chapter.

CHAPTER 10

Lung Disorders

I. CHRONIC OBSTRUCTIVE PULMONARY DISEASE (COPD)

Definition — a condition that results in a chronic obstruction to air flow within the lungs.

Diseases classified as COPD:
1. Emphysema
2. Chronic bronchitis
3. Asthma
4. Cystic fibrosis
5. Bronchiectasis

A. **Emphysema**
1. **Definition** — a permanent abnormal enlargement of the air spaces distal to the terminal bronchioles, which undergo destructive changes in the alveolar walls.
   a. Panlobular (panacinar) type — the entire lobule or gas exchange unit is affected
      (1) Acinus is the gas exchange unit of the lung, consisting of the respiratory bronchiole, alveolar duct, alveolar sacs, and the alveoli.
      (2) Entire acinus involved in this type of emphysema
      (3) Significant loss of lung parenchyma
      (4) Alveoli destroyed
      (5) Presence of bulla
      (6) Usually associated with emphysema resulting from $alpha_1$-antitrypsin deficiency
   b. Centrilobular (centriacinar) — the lesion is in the central portion of the lobule or gas exchange unit
      (1) Lesion in the center of the lobules results in enlargement and destruction of the respiratory bronchioles.
      (2) Usually involves the upper lung fields and is most commonly associated with chronic bronchitis
   c. Bullous emphysema
      (1) Emphysematous changes are isolated with the development of bulla.
      (2) **Bulla** is an air space more than 1 centimeter in diameter in its distended state.
      (3) **Bleb** is an air space adjacent to the pleura, usually less than 1 centimeter in diameter in its distended state.
2. **Etiology**
   a. Smoking
   b. $Alpha_1$-antitrypsin deficiency (hereditary).
3. **Pathophysiology**
   a. Elastic recoil of the lung is diminished, resulting in premature airway closure.
   b. Inspiratory flowrates are normal while expiratory flowrates are reduced.
   c. Air trapping leads to chronic hyperinflation

117

of the lungs and **increased functional residual capacity (FRC)**.

    d. **Lung compliance is increased** due to the loss of elastic lung tissue from the destructive process.

    e. Emphysema diminishes the area over which gas exchange occurs and is accompanied by regional differences in ventilation and perfusion. This accounts for increased physiologic dead space and the abnormal ABG values observed in emphysema patients.

4. **Clinical signs and symptoms**
   a. Dyspnea — initially on exertion; progressively worsens
   b. Digital clubbing — results from **chronic hypoxemia**
   c. Increased A-P chest diameter (barrel chest)
   d. Use of accessory muscles during normal breathing
   e. Elevated hemoglobin and hematocrit levels and red blood cell count
   f. Arterial blood gas measurements reveal chronic carbon dioxide retention and hypoxemia (advanced stages)
   g. Reduced breath sounds and hyperresonance to percussion
   h. Right-sided heart failure (cor pulmonale) in advanced stages
   i. Cyanosis

5. **X-ray characteristics**
   a. Flattened diaphragm
   b. Hyperinflation
   c. Reduced vascular markings
   d. Bullous lesions

6. **Pulmonary function studies**
   a. Increased residual volume and FRC
   b. Decreased diffusion capacity
   c. Decreased forced vital capacity (FVC)
   d. Decreased forced expiratory volume in 1 second (FEV_1) (decreased FEV_1/FVC)
   e. Prolonged nitrogen washout

7. **Treatment**
   a. Stop smoking
   b. Adequate hydration
   c. Postural drainage
   d. Bronchodilators
   e. Prevention of infections with immunizations
   f. Exercise (walking)
   g. Breathing exercise training
      (1) Diaphragmatic breathing exercises
      (2) **Pursed lip breathing** — prevents premature airway closure by producing

a back pressure into the airways on exhalation

    h. Care must be taken when administering oxygen to emphysema patients who chronically retain carbon dioxide and are chronically hypoxemic. Levels of Pa_{O_2} should be maintained at 50 to 60 torr to avoid knocking out the patient's "hypoxic drive."

NOTE: **If, after placing a severe COPD patient on oxygen, the Pa_{O_2} increases above 60 to 70 torr and the Pa_{CO_2} begins increasing, this should be recognized as knocking out the patient's hypoxic drive and the oxygen percentage should be decreased. Remember, maintain the Pa_{O_2} level at 50 to 60 torr.**

NOTE: **If the choice of which oxygen delivery device to use on a COPD patient is between a nasal cannula or a Venturi mask at approximately the same percentage, choose the Venturi mask.**

B. **Chronic bronchitis**
   1. **Definition** — chronic, excessive mucus production resulting from an increase in the number and size of mucous glands and goblet cells. It results in a cough and increased mucus production for at least 3 months of the year for more than 2 consecutive years.
   2. **Etiology**
      a. Smoking
      b. Males are most commonly affected.
   3. **Pathophysiology**
      a. Increase in the size of mucous glands
      b. Increase in the number of goblet cells
      c. Inflammation of bronchial walls
      d. Mucus plugs in peripheral airways
      e. Loss of cilia
      f. Emphysematous changes in advanced stages
      g. Narrowing airways leading to air flow obstruction
   4. **Clinical signs and symptoms**
      a. Cough with sputum production
      b. Dyspnea on exertion progressing to dyspnea with less effort
      c. Carbon dioxide retention and hypoxemia (advanced stages)
      d. Increased pulmonary vascular resistance (advanced stages)
      e. Increased hemoglobin, hematocrit, and RBC levels (advanced stages)
      f. Right-sided heart failure (cor pulmonale) in advanced stages
   5. **X-ray characteristics**
      a. Not significant in early disease
      b. Hyperinflation (advanced stages)

6. **Pulmonary function studies**
   a. Normal in early disease
   b. Increased residual volume
   c. Decreased FEV_1
   d. Decreased inspiratory flowrates in obstructive bronchitis
7. **Treatment**
   a. Identical to that for emphysema

C. **Asthma**

1. **Definition** — disease characterized by an increased reactivity of the trachea and bronchi to various stimuli, resulting in bronchoconstriction (bronchospasm), increased mucus production, and mucosal swelling.
2. **Etiology**
   a. **Extrinsic asthma (allergic asthma)**
      (1) Begins early in life
      (2) Caused by inhalation of airborne antigens (dust, pollen, etc.)
      (3) Exercise often precipitates bronchospasm
   b. **Intrinsic asthma (nonallergic asthma)**
      (1) Nonseasonal, nonallergic form of asthma occurring later in life
      (2) Caused by inhalation of pollutants (dust, fumes, smoke, etc.), infections, and emotional crisis
      (3) Usually a chronic, persistent form of asthma as opposed to the episodic nature of extrinsic asthma
3. **Pathophysiology**
   a. Mast cells in the bronchial tree are stimulated, causing the release of:
      (1) Histamine
      (2) Leukotrienes
      (3) Slow-reacting substance of anaphylaxis (SRS-A)
      (4) Eosinophilic chemotactic factor of anaphylaxis (ECF-A)
      (5) Prostaglandins
   b. The release of these substances results in:
      (1) Bronchoconstriction
      (2) Mucosal edema
      (3) Increased mucus production
      (4) Accumulation of eosinophils in the blood
      (5) Vasodilation
4. **Clinical signs and symptoms**
   a. Mild wheezing and cough initially; may progress to severe dyspnea if the attack is not arrested
   b. Cough is initially nonproductive, progressing to productive by the end of the episode.

c. Secretions reveal high eosinophil levels.
   d. Intercostal and supraclavicular retractions
   e. Use of accessory muscles to breathe (severe attack)
   f. Paradoxical pulse — systolic blood pressure is 10 mm Hg higher on expiration than on inspiration
   g. Tachycardia and tachypnea
   h. ABG measurements initially reveal hypoxemia and low Pa_{CO_2}. (Pa_{CO_2} will increase as attack worsens.)
   i. Cyanosis
5. **X-ray characteristics**
   a. Hyperinflation (hyperlucency of lung fields)
   b. Atelectasis — less common
   c. Infiltrates
6. **Pulmonary function studies**
   a. Decreased FEV_1
   b. Decreased FVC
   c. Decreased FEV_1/FVC
   d. Increased residual volume
7. **Treatment (preventive)**
   a. Prevention
      (1) Avoid known allergens or causative factors
   b. Medications
      (1) Bronchodilators
      (2) Cromolyn sodium — **prevents attacks by stabilizing the mast cell. Not used during an attack.**
      (3) Corticosteroids
      (4) Anticholinergic drugs (atropine)
8. **Treatment (during an attack)**
   a. Bronchodilators
   b. Intravenous fluids
   c. Oxygen therapy
   d. Intravenous aminophylline
9. **Status asthmaticus** — severe asthmatic attack not responding to treatment with an adequate amount of routine medications within a few hours.
   a. Patient should be hospitalized immediately.
   b. Intravenous aminophylline
   c. Hydration
   d. Intravenous corticosteroids
   e. Supplemental oxygen
   f. Close monitoring of ABG values and oxygen saturation
   g. Bronchodilators
   h. Chest physiotherapy (if tolerated) to remove mucous plugs and secretions
   i. If not controlled, intubate and institute mechanical ventilation.

D. **Cystic fibrosis (mucoviscidosis)**
   1. **Definition** — a hereditary disease affecting the exocrine glands of the body that results in production of abnormally thick secretions by these glands. The glands most commonly affected are located in the pancreas, the sweat glands, and the respiratory system.
   2. **Etiology**
      a. Genetically transmitted
      b. Both mother and father must be carriers of the autosomal recessive gene. With each pregnancy there is a one out of four chance the child will have the disease.
   3. **Pathophysiology**
      a. The abnormally high numbers of goblet cells and bronchial glands located in the tracheo-bronchial tree secrete large amounts of thick, tenacious mucus.
      b. Because the mucus is so thick, it stagnates in the airways, leading to airway obstruction and facilitating growth of bacteria.
      c. Mucus plugging leads to atelectasis, hyper-inflation, and pneumonia.
      d. Abnormalities in the pancreatic ducts and glands lead to inadequate absorption and digestion of food, causing malnutrition if not properly treated.
   4. **Clinical signs and symptoms**
      a. Cough
      b. Tachycardia and tachypnea
      c. Increased A-P chest diameter
      d. Production of thick, tenacious mucus
      e. Digital clubbing
      f. Use of accessory muscles during quiet breathing
      g. Acute alveolar hyperventilation with hypox-emia in early stages
      h. Chronic ventilatory failure with hypoxemia in the late stages
      i. Cyanosis
      j. Cor pulmonale in late stages
      k. Elevated sweat chloride levels
   5. **X-ray characteristics**
      a. Hyperinflation
      b. Flattened diaphragm
      c. Increased lung markings
      d. Cardiomegaly
   6. **Pulmonary function studies**
      a. Decreased FVC
      b. Decreased FEV_1
      c. Decreased FEV_1/FVC ratio
      d. Increased FRC and RV
   7. **Treatment**
      a. Postural drainage and percussion

   b. Bronchodilator therapy
   c. Mucolytics — Mucomyst (acetylcysteine)
   c. Oxygen therapy
   d. Antibiotics
   e. Aerosol therapy
   f. Expectorants

E. **Bronchiectasis**
   1. **Definition** — a chronic dilation of the bronchi and bronchioles that results in inflammation and damage to the walls of these airways
   2. **Etiology**
      a. Chronic respiratory infections
      b. Tuberculosis lesion
      c. Patients with cystic fibrosis
      d. Bronchial obstruction
   3. **Pathophysiology**
      a. It is not clear whether the chronic dilation is a result of destructive changes in the bron-chial walls owing to inflammation and infection or a result of a congenital defect of the airways.
      b. Bronchial obstruction may render the mucociliary transport system ineffective, leading to an accumulation of thick secre-tions.
      c. The bronchial wall is destroyed, with a resultant atrophy of the mucosal layer.
   4. **Clinical signs and symptoms**
      a. Productive cough with large amounts of thick, purulent secretions that may be foul smelling
      b. Tachypnea and tachycardia
      c. Hemoptysis
      d. Recurrent pulmonary infections
      e. Digital clubbing
      f. Cyanosis
      g. Respiratory alkalosis with hypoxemia (early stage)
      h. Chronic respiratory acidosis with hypoxemia (late stage)
      i. Barrel chest
   5. **X-ray characteristics**
      a. Increased lung markings
      b. Flattened diaphragm
      c. Segmental atelectasis
   6. **Pulmonary function studies**
      a. Decreased FVC
      b. Decreased FRC
      c. Decreased FEV_1
      d. Decreased $FEF_{25\%}$ to $FEF_{75\%}$

Because of the decreased values in both flows and volumes, this disease may be both obstructive and restrictive.

7. **Treatment**
   a. Chest physical therapy
   b. Aerosol therapy
   c. Bronchodilator therapy
   d. Mucolytics — Mucomyst
   e. Antibiotics
   f. Oxygen therapy
   g. Expectorants

II. LOWER RESPIRATORY TRACT INFECTIONS

A. **Pneumonia**
   1. **Definition** — acute inflammation of the gas exchange units of the lungs.
   2. **Etiology**
      a. Various organisms (discussed later in this section)
      b. Decreased airway defense mechanisms due to:
         (1) Ineffective cough
         (2) Obtunded airway reflexes
         (3) Impaired mucociliary transport system
         (4) Obstructed airways
      c. Various conditions result in predisposition to pneumonia
         (1) COPD
         (2) Alcoholism
         (3) Malnutrition
         (4) Seizure disorders
         (5) Chronic debilitating illnesses
         (6) Major surgical procedures
         (7) Old age
   3. **Pathophysiology**
      a. Pathogenic microorganisms that reach the gas exchange areas of the lung cause an intense tissue reaction resulting in production of inflammatory exudates and cells.
      b. The white blood cells (WBCs) phagocytize the invading organisms, leading to further inflammation.
      c. As the lungs begin filling with the inflammatory exudates and cells, they become **consolidated.**
      d. If tissue necrosis is not present, the lung will heal and return to normal function.
      e. If necrosis occurs, healing is slow, with production of fibrous scar tissue and loss of normal lung function.
   4. **Clinical signs and symptoms**
      a. Infection
      b. Malaise
      c. Fever
      d. Chest pain
      e. Dyspnea and tachycardia
      f. Inspiratory crackles on auscultation
   5. **X-ray characteristics**
      a. Consolidation
      b. Air bronchogram
   6. **Types of pneumonia**
      a. Bacterial
         (1) *Streptococcus pneumoniae* (pneumococcal pneumonia) — **most common bacterial pneumonia**
         (2) *Haemophilus influenzae*
         (3) *Klebsiella pneumoniae*
         (4) *Legionella pneumoniae*
         (5) *Pseudomonas aeruginosa*
      b. *Mycoplasma pneumoniae* — smaller than bacteria and more common in children
      c. Viral
         (1) Influenza
         (2) Adenovirus
         (3) Chickenpox
      d. Protozoan
         (1) *Pneumocystis carinii* pneumonia (PCP)
            (a) Pneumonia commonly seen in patients with acquired immunodeficiency syndrome (AIDS)
            (b) This severe complication is diagnosed in about 60% of AIDS cases.
            (c) Definitive diagnosis is made from cultures of lung secretions and lung tissue
            (d) *P. carinii* is commonly treated with the anti-protozoan drug **pentamidine** via aerosolization.
   7. **Treatment**
      a. Antibiotics
      b. Supplemental oxygen
      c. Chest physiotherapy
      d. Adequate hydration
      e. Adequate nutrition
      f. Tracheal suctioning (if poor removal of secretions due to ineffective cough)

B. **Lung abscess**
   1. **Definition** — an infection of the lung characterized by a localized accumulation of pus with destruction of the surrounding tissue.
   2. **Etiology**
      a. Most commonly caused by anaerobic bacteria
      b. Aerobic bacteria, including staphylococci, streptococci, and some gram-negative bacteria, may be less common causes

c. May follow aspiration

d. Associated with lung cancer

3. **Pathophysiology**

a. In the acute phase, it resembles pneumonia.

b. As progression occurs, necrosis is evident and may spread to adjacent lung tissue.

4. **Clinical signs and symptoms**

a. Fever

b. Productive cough (initially nonproductive or minimal production followed by production of **purulent, foul-smelling secretions**)

c. Chest pain

d. Weight loss

e. Hemoptysis

f. Digital clubbing

g. Tachycardia

h. Tachypnea

5. **X-ray characteristics**

a. Localized area of consolidation

b. Most common sites include the superior segments of lower lobes and posterior segments of upper lobes (due to position during an aspiration event)

6. **Laboratory findings**

a. Increased WBC count

b. Anemia (decreased RBC count)

c. Sputum culture reveals pus cells and necrotic material

7. **Treatment**

a. Antibiotics

b. Postural drainage

c. Adequate nutrition

NOTE: If an abscess ruptures into the pleura, pus will accumulate in the pleural space. This is an empyema and should be drained prior to chest physiotherapy.

C. Tuberculosis (TB)

1. **Definition** — A granulomatous bacterial infection, chronic in nature, affecting the lungs and other organs of the body

2. **Etiology** — Caused by the inhalation or ingestion of the bacteria, *Mycobacterium tuberculosis*. These organisms are known as **acid-fast bacilli** and are usually spread through coughing and sneezing. Diagnosis is obtained from skin tests, chest x-ray, and sputum culture showing the presence of acid-fast bacilli.

3. **Pathophysiology**

a. After the bacillus is inhaled it enters the alveoli, resulting in an inflammatory reaction similar to that seen with pneumonia (discussed earlier in this chapter).

b. Macrophages enter the infected area and engulf the bacilli without fully killing them.

c. The lung tissue surrounding this area encapsulates the bacilli, providing a protective covering. This is called a granuloma or tubercle.

d. The granuloma fills with necrotic material and is referred to as a caseous (cheese-like) granuloma.

e. If the patient's immunologic system controls this process or if antituberculosis drugs are given, the lung tissue will fibrose and calcify as healing occurs. This may result in a stiffness or decreased lung compliance in the affected area.

f. In most cases, the patient's own immunologic mechanisms keep the bacilli in check, but the organisms will remain dormant in the lungs for many years, resulting in a positive TB skin test. These encapsulated bacilli can escape in later years, causing infection.

g. Chronic dilation of the bronchi (bronchiectasis) may result during the healing process of TB.

h. In uncontrolled cases, the tubercles increase in size and combine to form larger tubercles, which may rupture, permitting air and the infected material to enter the pleural space and bronchi and bronchioles.

NOTE: It is important to note that most individuals infected with the TB bacteria often have little if any symptoms. The primary TB lesion heals completely, possibly leaving a small scar, which could calcify later in life.

4. **Clinical signs and symptoms**

a. Cough

b. Sputum production — positive for acid-fast bacilli

c. Tachycardia

d. Increased cardiac output

e. Chest pain

f. Hemoptysis

g. Dull percussion note

h. Rales and rhonchi

i. Hyperventilation and hypoxemia (early stages)

j. Chronic respiratory acidosis with hypoxemia (late stages)

k. Cyanosis (severe cases)

5. **X-ray characteristics**

a. Enlarged lymph nodes in hilar region (lymphadenopathy)
b. Pleural effusion
c. Cavitation
d. Ghon complex (lung lesions and lymph node involvement)
e. Fibrosis
f. Infiltrates

6. **Pulmonary function studies**
   a. Decreased vital capacity
   b. Decreased functional residual capacity
   c. Decreased residual volume
   d. Decreased total lung capacity

NOTE: These PFT findings are characteristic of the restrictive lung processes that occur in tuberculosis.

7. Treatment
   a. Supplemental oxygen
   b. Antituberculosis drugs
      (1) Rifampin
      (2) Isoniazid (INH)
      (3) Ethambutol
      (4) Streptomycin

NOTE: These drugs are used in combination for 2 to 4 months.

   c. Placement in respiratory isolation
   d. Routine airway maintenance

III. OTHER LUNG DISORDERS

A. **Pulmonary edema (cardiogenic)**
   1. **Definition** — excessive amount of fluid in the lung tissues and/or alveoli due to an increase in pulmonary capillary pressure resulting from abnormal left heart function
   2. **Etiology**
      a. Left heart failure
      b. Aortic stenosis
      c. Mitral valve stenosis
      d. Systemic hypertension
      NOTE: These four causes result in the backup of fluid from the heart into the pulmonary capillaries, which become engorged, leading to pulmonary edema.
      e. Alveolar capillary membrane leak due to injury, such as that seen in ARDS (non-cardiogenic pulmonary edema)
   3. **Pathophysiology**
      a. Fluid is maintained within the capillaries by two forces:

      (1) **Plasma oncotic pressure** (to keep fluid in the capillaries)
      (2) **Capillary hydrostatic pressure** (to push fluid out of the capillaries)
      b. Oncotic pressure is normally much higher than capillary hydrostatic pressure, keeping fluid in the capillaries.
      c. As fluid from the heart backs up into the pulmonary circulation, capillary hydrostatic pressure increases above plasma oncotic pressure and fluid leaks into the interstitial spaces.
      d. Excess fluid overwhelms the lymphatics (which normally drain the interstitial spaces) and drains into the alveoli, resulting in **decreased lung compliance.**
      e. Airway resistance increases due to excess fluid.
      f. Widened P(A–a) gradient results from intrapulmonary shunting and ventilation/perfusion mismatch.
   4. **Clinical signs and symptoms**
      a. Dyspnea
         (1) **Orthopnea** — dyspnea while reclining (relieved by sitting upright in semi-Fowler's or Fowler's position)
         (2) **Paroxysmal nocturnal dyspnea** — severe attack of dyspnea during sleep that awakes the patient (relieved by sitting up in semi-Fowler's position)
      b. Productive cough with thin, pink, frothy secretions
      c. Rales auscultated in bases (all lung fields in severe edema)
      d. Tachypnea
      e. Cyanosis
      f. Diaphoresis — sweating
      g. Distended neck veins
      h. Tachycardia or other arrhythmias
   5. **X-ray characteristics**
      a. Increased vascular markings
      b. Interstitial edema
      c. Enlarged heart shadow
   6. **Treatment**
      a. Oxygen administration (percentage based on Pa_{O_2})
      b. Cardiac glycosides
      c. Ventilatory support with PEEP (if severe)
      d. Adequate airway maintenance
      e. Morphine
      f. IPPB with ethyl alcohol (40% to 50%)
B. **Pulmonary embolism**
   1. **Definition** — obstruction of the pulmonary artery or one of its branches by a blood clot

a. **Embolus** — a clot that travels through the bloodstream from another vessel and lodges in a smaller one, thus obstructing blood flow

2. **Etiology**
   a. The blood clot usually originates in deep veins of the legs or pelvic area, dislodges, travels back to the heart through the venous system, and lodges in the pulmonary artery.
   b. Clot originally forms due to stagnation or venous stasis from prolonged bed rest, immobility due to pain of trauma or surgery, or paralysis.
   c. Seen in COPD patients due to venous stasis resulting from the increased viscosity of their blood (increased RBC)

3. **Pathophysiology**
   a. Blood flow is obstructed to areas of the involved lung, contributing to dead space ventilation (ventilation without perfusion).
   b. Lung compliance decreases.
   c. Widened $P(A–a)$ gradient results from intrapulmonary shunting and ventilation/perfusion mismatch.
   d. Lung volumes decrease.

4. **Clinical signs and symptoms**
   a. Dyspnea
   b. Chest pain
   c. Tachypnea
   d. Cough
   e. Pleuritic pain
   f. Hemoptysis
   g. Tenderness and swelling in lower extremities due to thrombophlebitis
   h. Tachycardia
   i. Cyanosis
   j. Decreased breath sounds over the affected area (wheezing and rales may be heard)

5. **X-ray characteristics**
   a. May be normal
   b. Decreased lung volume
   c. Linear densities of atelectasis
   d. Pleural effusion
   e. Elevated hemidiaphragm

6. **Treatment**
   a. Prevention
      (1) Use of elastic stockings
      (2) Proper positioning
      (3) Ambulation
   b. Anticoagulation therapy
   c. Supplemental oxygen

C. **Acute respiratory distress syndrome (ARDS)**
   1. **Definition** — a group of symptoms causing acute respiratory failure resulting from pulmonary injury from various causes

2. **Etiology**
   a. Diffuse lung injury
      (1) Sepsis
      (2) Aspiration
      (3) Near drowning
      (4) Oxygen toxicity
      (5) Shock
      (6) Thoracic trauma
      (7) Extensive burn
      (8) Inhalation of toxic gases
      (9) Fluid overload
      (10) Fat embolism
      (11) Narcotic overdose
   b. Most patients have no previous pulmonary problems.

3. **Pathophysiology**
   a. Lung injury precedes an inflammatory process.
   b. Alveolar capillary membrane begins to leak, causing noncardiogenic pulmonary edema.
   c. Fluid builds up in the interstitial spaces, alveoli, and distal airways.
   d. Surfactant production decreases and atelectasis results, accompanied by excessive fluid in the alveoli and airways.
   e. Because of inflammatory cells, fibrin, and cellular debris from the inflammatory process, the lungs become stiff and lung compliance decreases.
   f. In severe cases, the lungs may become almost entirely atelectatic, leading to large intrapulmonary shunting.

4. **Clinical signs and symptoms**
   a. Hypoxemia — refractory (not responsive) to oxygen therapy in severe cases
   b. Cyanosis
   c. Severe dyspnea and cough
   d. Decreased lung compliance
   e. Suprasternal and intercostal retractions
   f. Widened $P(A–a)$ gradient on 100% oxygen (severe cases)
   g. Tachypnea

5. **X-ray characteristics**
   a. Interstitial edema
   b. Alveolar edema (fluffy infiltration)

6. **Treatment**
   a. Usually not managed well on high oxygen concentrations alone due to decreased lung compliance
   b. Mechanical ventilation with **PEEP**
      (1) Because the lungs are noncompliant, peak inspiratory pressures are markedly elevated.

(2) Add PEEP if Pa$_{O_2}$ is below normal on an F$_{IO_2}$ of 0.60 or greater.

  c. Monitor heart pressures (PAP, PCWP) with Swan-Ganz catheter

  d. Diuretics

  e. Routine airway maintenance

D. **Pneumothorax**

  1. **Definition** — the presence of air in the pleural space

  2. **Etiology**

    a. Spontaneous pneumothorax

      (1) Develops without trauma

      (2) Seen most commonly in tall, thin, young males due to bleb rupture

      (3) Seen in COPD patients due to bullous disease and bleb rupture

    b. Traumatic pneumothorax

      (1) Broken ribs

      (2) Puncture wound

      (3) Chest or neck surgery

  3. **Pathophysiology**

    a. Negative pressure is normally present in the pleural space. Any communication between the atmosphere and pleural space will draw air into the space, causing the lung to collapse.

    b. The volume of the unaffected lung will increase along with perfusion by more blood, which helps prevent severe hypoxemia.

    c. **Tension pneumothorax** occurs if the opening in the lung to the pleural space acts as a one-way valve permitting air to enter the space but not allowing the air to exit.

      (1) Ventilation of the affected lung diminishes.

      (2) The trapped air increases pressure on the affected side, pushing the trachea and mediastinum to the unaffected side.

      (3) The **immediate action** to take is to relieve the pressure in the pleural space by inserting a needle in the second or third intercostal space.

  4. **Clinical signs and symptoms**

    a. Chest pain

    b. Dyspnea

    c. Decreased breath sounds over affected lung

    d. Hyperresonant percussion note over affected lung

    e. Asymmetrical chest excursion

    f. Tachypnea (severe cases)

    g. Cyanosis (severe cases)

  5. **X-ray characteristics**

    a. Hyperlucency

    b. Deviation of heart, trachea, and mediastinum to the opposite (unaffected) side if tension pneumothorax is present

  6. **Treatment**

    a. Needle aspiration — **immediate if tension pneumothorax**

    b. Placement of chest tube

    c. Supplemental oxygen as needed (monitor oxygen saturation or ABG values)

E. **Pleural effusion**

  1. **Definition** — excessive fluid in the pleural space

    a. Transudate — fluid caused by an imbalance between transcapillary pressure and plasma oncotic pressure

    b. Exudate — fluid caused by increased capillary permeability, as in inflammation

  2. **Etiology**

    a. Transudative pleural effusion

      (1) Congestive heart failure (most common)

      (2) Cirrhosis of the liver

      (3) Kidney disease

    b. Exudative pleural effusion

      (1) Infections

      (2) Trauma

      (3) Surgery

      (4) Tumors

      (5) Pulmonary embolism

  3. **Pathophysiology**

    a. Fluid accumulates in the pleural space because of an imbalance between formation and absorption of the fluid.

    b. Increased fluid formation may cause pleural effusion.

    c. Decreased absorption may cause pleural effusion.

  4. **Clinical signs and symptoms**

    a. Chest pain

    b. Dyspnea

    c. Dullness to percussion

    d. Absent breath sounds over the fluid

  5. **X-ray characteristics**

    a. Blunting of costophrenic angle

    b. Homogeneous density in dependent part of the hemithorax

NOTE: For small effusions, a lateral decubitus x-ray should be taken.

  6. **Treatment**

    a. Drain fluid by thoracentesis

    b. Chest tube drainage may be necessary in chronic cases.

    c. Supplemental oxygen as needed (monitor ABG values or oxygen saturation)

IV. SLEEP APNEA

A. Sleep apnea is diagnosed in patients with at least 30 episodes of apnea over a 6-hour period of sleep.
B. The apneic period may last from 20 seconds to 1.5 minutes.
C. **Types of sleep apnea**
   1. **Obstructive sleep apnea**
      a. Apnea due to anatomic obstruction of upper airway
      b. During the apneic period, the patient exhibits **strong and often intense respiratory effort.**
      c. Although sleep posture (sleeping on side rather than supine) has some benefits, **the use of CPAP while sleeping is the most effective treatment for obstructive sleep apnea.**
      d. Obstructive sleep apnea may be associated with
         (1) Obesity
         (2) Excessive pharyngeal tissue
         (3) Deviated nasal septum
         (4) Laryngeal web
         (5) Laryngeal stenosis
         (6) Enlarged adenoids or tonsils
      e. **Symptoms of obstructive sleep apnea**
         (1) Loud snoring
         (2) Hypersomnolence (excessive daytime sleeping)
         (3) Morning headache
         (4) Nausea
         (5) Personality changes
   2. **Central sleep apnea**
      a. Apnea occurs due to the failure of the central respiratory centers (medulla, pons) to send signals to the respiratory muscles.
      b. **Characterized by the absence of inspiratory effort with no diaphragmatic movement (unlike obstructive sleep apnea)**
      c. Associated with central nervous system disorders

   d. Central sleep apnea may also be associated with
      (1) Hypoventilation syndrome
      (2) Encephalitis
      (3) Spinal surgery
      (4) Brainstem disorders
   e. **Symptoms of central sleep apnea**
      (1) Insomnia
      (2) Mild snoring
      (3) Depression
      (4) Fatigue during the day

NOTE: Some patients may have a combination of obstructive and central sleep apnea known as mixed sleep apnea.

REFERENCES

Des Jardins T. *Clinical Manifestations of Respiratory Disease.* 2nd ed. Chicago: Year Book Medical Publishers; 1990.
Farzan S. *A Concise Handbook of Respiratory Diseases.* 3rd ed. Norwalk, CT: Appleton & Lange; 1992.
Mitchell R, Petty T. *Synopsis of Clinical Pulmonary Disease.* 3rd ed. St. Louis: CV Mosby; 1982.

PRETEST ANSWERS

1. D
2. D
3. B
4. B
5. A
6. C

▼▼ Respiratory Medications

PRETEST QUESTIONS*

1. Which of the following is frequently used with aerosol therapy to promote coughing?

A. normal saline
B. hypotonic saline
C. hypertonic saline
D. propylene glycol

2. If cromolyn sodium is given during an acute asthma attack, you should expect

A. brochodilation to occur with relief of dyspnea.
B. the respiratory rate to decrease.
C. no change in symptoms.
D. patient response within 1 hour.

3. To improve the mobilization of thick, inspissated secretions, which medication would be of most benefit?

A. acetylcysteine (Mucomyst)
B. normal saline
C. sterile water
D. hypotonic saline

4. With which of these medications would you be concerned about heart rate changes?

  I. propylene glycol
 II. metaproterenol (Alupent, Metaprel)
III. hypotonic saline
IV. terbutaline sulfate (Brethine, Bricanyl)

A. I only
B. I and II only
C. II and III only
D. II and IV only

5. Which of the following medications would be of most benefit in the treatment of a patient with post-extubation stridor?

A. hypotonic saline
B. acetylcysteine (Mucomyst)
C. pancuronium bromide (Pavulon)
D. racemic epinephrine (microNefrin, Vaponefrin)

*See answers at the end of the chapter.

Respiratory Medications

I. CLASSIFICATION OF RESPIRATORY MEDICATIONS

A. **Diluents**
1. **Normal saline (0.9% sodium chloride [NaCl])**
   a. Used to dilute bronchodilators
   b. Used to dilute secretions for improved expectoration; often instilled 3 to 5 ml at a time through E-T tubes and tracheostomy tubes prior to suctioning
2. **Hypotonic saline (0.4% NaCl)**
   a. Used in ultrasonic nebulizers because lower concentration produces smaller particles
   b. More stable than sterile water
3. **Hypertonic saline (1.8% NaCl)**
   a. Larger aerosol particles are produced due to higher solution concentration.
   b. Used to stimulate coughing and induce sputum by irritation of the airway
4. **Sterile distilled water**
   a. Used to dilute other medications
   b. Used to hydrate secretions, thereby decreasing viscosity for easier expectoration
   c. Used to humidify dry gases
B. **Mucolytics** — drugs that break sputum down chemically for more effective expectoration
1. **Acetylcysteine (Mucomyst)**

a. Available in 10% or 20% solutions
b. Breaks the **disulfide bonds** in the sputum, which decreases viscosity
c. Often used with bronchodilators, as **bronchospasm** is a common side effect
d. Should be used in patients with **thick secretions that are difficult to mobilize**
e. Often used in patients with cystic fibrosis or bronchiectasis
f. May be nebulized (1 to 3 ml t.i.d. or q.i.d.) or instilled directly into the trachea
g. Should bronchospasm occur, stop the treatment immediately and administer a bronchodilator.
h. Irritating to oral mucosal tissues — patient should rinse mouth after treatment
2. **Sodium bicarbonate (2% NaHCO$_3$)**
   a. Increases sputum pH, thereby decreasing its viscosity
   b. May be used to improve the mucolytic actions of acetylcysteine
   c. Dosage: 2 to 5 ml via aerosol or 2 to 10 ml instilled directly into the trachea every 4 to 8 hours
C. **Sympathomimetic bronchodilators**

NOTE: **These medications stimulate one or more of the following receptors:**

Receptor	Location	Response
Alpha	Mucosal blood vessels; bronchial smooth muscle	Vasoconstriction; bronchoconstriction
Beta$_1$	Heart muscle	Increase in heart rate and cardiac output; arrhythmias
Beta$_2$	Bronchial smooth muscle; peripheral mucosal blood vessels; CNS and peripheral limb muscles	Bronchodilation; vasodilation; nervousness (CNS); tingling in fingers

NOTE: The ideal bronchodilator is a pure beta$_2$-receptor stimulator.

1. **Epinephrine (Adrenalin, Sus-Phrine)**
   a. Stimulates all three receptors (beta$_1$ most affected)
   b. Duration of action is 0.5 to 2 hours.
   c. Used to stimulate the heart — not commonly used as a bronchodilator
   d. Adverse effects:
      (1) Increased heart rate
      (2) Hypertension
      (3) Anxiety
      (4) Mild bronchoconstriction
   e. Dosage: As an aerosol, 0.1 to 0.5 ml (1:100) in 3 to 5 ml of diluent
2. **Racemic epinephrine (microNefrin, Vaponefrin)**
   a. Stimulates all three receptors (beta$_1$ most affected)
   b. Duration of action is 0.5 to 2 hours.
   c. Used to decrease mucosal edema and inflammation after extubation or in pediatric patients with croup
   d. Has milder effects than epinephrine (one-half strength)
   e. Dosage: As an aerosol, 0.2 to 0.5 ml in 3 to 5 ml of diluent every 3 to 4 hours
3. **Isoetharine (Bronkosol)**
   a. Stimulates beta$_1$ and beta$_2$ receptors
   b. Duration of action is 1 to 4 hours.
   c. Used to decrease airway resistance
   d. Adverse effects
      (1) Increased heart rate
      (2) Increased blood pressure
      (3) Anxiety
      (4) Paresthesia
      (5) Dizziness
   e. Dosage: 0.25 to 0.5 ml in 3 to 5 ml of diluent t.i.d. or q.i.d.
4. **Isoproterenol (Isuprel)**
   a. Strong beta$_1$ and beta$_2$ stimulator
   b. Duration of action is 1 to 2 hours.

   c. Used to decrease airway resistance
   d. Adverse effects
      (1) Increased heart rate
      (2) Increased blood pressure
      (3) Anxiety
      (4) Tingling in fingers
      (5) Nervousness
   e. Dosage: 0.25 to 0.5 ml in 3 to 5 ml of diluent t.i.d. or q.i.d.
5. **Metaproterenol (Alupent, Metaprel)**
   a. Very minor beta$_1$ and mild beta$_2$ stimulator
   b. Duration of action is 4 to 6 hours.
   c. Used to decrease airway resistance
   d. Adverse effects
      (1) Mild cardiac effects
      (2) Mild CNS effects
   e. Dosage: 0.1 to 0.3 ml in 3 to 5 ml of diluent every 4 hours
6. **Terbutaline sulfate (Brethine, Bricanyl)**
   a. **Very minor beta$_1$** and **moderate beta$_2$** stimulator
   b. Duration of action is 3 to 7 hours.
   c. Used to decrease airway resistance
   d. Adverse effects
      (1) Mild cardiac effects
      (2) Mild CNS effects
   e. Dosage: 0.25 to 0.5 mg in 3 to 5 ml of diluent every 4 to 8 hours
7. **Albuterol (Proventil, Ventolin)**
   a. **Mild beta$_1$** and **strong beta$_2$** stimulator
   b. Duration of action is 4 to 6 hours.
   c. Used to decrease airway resistance
   d. Adverse effects
      (1) Mild cardiac effects
      (2) Mild CNS effects
   e. Dosage: 0.1 to 0.2 mg in 3 to 5 ml of diluent every 6 to 8 hours
D. **Parasympatholytic bronchodilators**
   1. **Atropine sulfate**
      a. An anticholinergic drug that blocks the cholinergic constricting influences on the airway and potentiates the adrenergic influences (beta$_2$ stimulation), resulting in bronchodilation
      b. Also inhibits secretion production and increases secretion viscosity

NOTE: There is more potential for mucus plugging in patients with thick secretions who are administered atropine systemically. Given as an aerosol, atropine has little effect on lung secretions but may dry out the oral mucosa.

   c. Used to decrease airway resistance, congestion, and cardiac arrhythmias

d. Adverse effects
   (1) Increased secretion viscosity
   (2) Dry mouth
   (3) CNS stimulation
e. Dosage: 1 mg in 3 to 5 ml of diluent every 4 to 6 hours

2. **Ipratropium bromide (Atrovent)**
  a. An anticholinergic bronchodilator that acts topically in the lung instead of systemically, as most bronchodilators do
  b. Duration of action is 3 to 4 hours.
  c. Used to decrease airway resistance, especially in asthmatics
  d. Adverse effects
    (1) Palpitations
    (2) Nervousness
    (3) Dizziness
    (4) Nausea
    (5) Tremors
  e. Dosage: Two inhalations (36 mcg) from metered-dose inhaler four times per day.

E. **Phosphodiesterase inhibitors**
1. These drugs are called **xanthines.** They inhibit the cellular production of phosphodiesterase, an enzyme that readily breaks down cyclic adenosine monophosphate (AMP), another cellular enzyme that produces bronchodilation. Lower amounts of phosphodiesterase allow increased production of cyclic AMP, thus increasing bronchodilation.
  a. **Theophylline (aminophylline)**
    (1) Stimulates respiratory rate and depth of breathing and produces pulmonary vasodilation and bronchodilation
    (2) Used to decrease airway resistance, especially in asthmatics
    (3) Duration of action is 4 to 6 hours.
    (4) Adverse effects
      (a) Cardiac effects
      (b) CNS effects
      (c) Nausea and vomiting
      (d) Diuresis
    (5) Dosage: Intravenous (IV) loading dose — 6 mg/kg; maintenance dose — 0.5 mg/kg/hr; average dose — 250 mg every 6 hours

NOTE: Therapeutic serum level is 10 to 20 mg/L.

F. **Miscellaneous respiratory drugs**
1. **Cromolyn sodium (Intal)**
  a. Stabilizes the mast cell, making it less sensitive to specific antigens and inhibiting the release of histamine

b. Duration of action is 2 to 6 hours.
c. Used as **preventive therapy** for asthma (**not effective during an asthma attack**)
d. Adverse effects:
   (1) Bronchospasm (when delivered in powder form)
   (2) Cough (powder form)
   (3) Local irritation (powder form)

NOTE: **Cromolyn sodium is now available in aerosolized form and is tolerated much better than in the powdered form. The powdered form was delivered through a device called a spinhaler. The capsule was punctured and placed in the device and the patient inhaled deeply, thus delivering the powder into the airway. Bronchospasm is a common complication when Intal is delivered in this form.**

  e. Dosage: one capsule (20 mg) q.i.d. (powder form); 20 mg q.i.d. (nebulized form)
2. **Ethanol (ethyl alcohol)**
  a. Used as an antifoam agent to decrease the surface tension of frothy, bubbly secretions observed with pulmonary edema
  b. Used in the treatment of pulmonary edema to disperse the edema bubbles, making the airway more patent
  c. Adverse effects
    (1) Mucosal irritation
    (2) Dry mouth
  d. Dosage: 3 to 15 ml of a 40% to 50% solution

G. **Neuromuscular blocking agents**
1. **Succinylcholine (Anectine)**
  a. A depolarizing agent that competes with acetylcholine for cholinergic receptors of the motor end plate of a muscle. If these receptors remain occupied by the depolarizing agent, further stimulation cannot occur and paralysis persists.
  b. Onset of action is in 1 minute with a duration of action of only **5 minutes.**
  c. Used as a short-term paralyzing agent to facilitate endotracheal intubation
  d. Adverse effects
    (1) Decreased heart rate
    (2) Decreased blood pressure
    NOTE: **Atropine may be administered to counteract this agent.**
  e. Dosage: 20 mg IV (2 to 3 mg/min)
2. **Tubocurarine (curare)**
  a. Nondepolarizing agent that blocks the transmission of acetylcholine at the postjunctional membrane

b. Onset of action is in 3 to 5 minutes with a duration of action of 40 to 90 minutes.

c. Used to paralyze patients who are resisting mechanical ventilation

d. Adverse effects
   (1) Bronchospasm (due to histamine release)
   (2) Decreased blood pressure

e. Dosage 2 to 3 mg every 45 to 60 minutes

3. Pancuronium bromide (Pavulon)
   a. Nondepolarizing agent that is five times stronger than curare and much more commonly used
   b. Onset of action is in 2 to 3 minutes with a duration of action of up to 1 hour
   c. Used to paralyze patients who are resisting mechanical ventilation
   d. Adverse effects
      (1) Increased heart rate (mild)
      (2) Increased blood pressure (mild)

NOTE: Unlike curare, pancuronium bromide does not cause the release of histamine; therefore, bronchospasm is not a problem.

e. Dosage: 4 to 5 mg IV in intervals of 1 to 3 hours

NOTE: The paralyzing effects of the nondepolarizing agents (curare and pancuronium bromide) may be reversed with the administration of neostigmine (Prostigmin) or edrophonium chloride (Tensilon).

H. Corticosteroids (aerosolized)

NOTE: These anti-inflammatory agents are used in respiratory care to prevent or reduce airway inflammation in asthma and upper airway swelling which accompanies glottic edema. Administering these agents via aerosol (usually metered-dose inhaler) reduces the systemic side effects such as the cushingoid symptoms (edema, moon facies) and adrenal suppression.

1. Dexamethasone sodium phosphate (Decadron)
   a. One of the first steroids administered successfully as an aerosol
   b. May be administered in metered-dose inhalers (MDI) or in aerosol solution
   c. Systemic side effects are common even when delivered via aerosol.

2. Beclomethasone dipropionate (Vanceril, Beclovent)
   a. Commonly used in asthma and other chronic lung diseases
   b. Fewer systemic side effects than Decadron
   c. Delivered by MDI

3. Flunisolide (AeroBid)
   a. Effective treatment for asthmatics
   b. Delivered by MDI

NOTE: Patients on MDI steroid therapy must be educated in the proper use of the MDI and possible side effects of the drugs if overused, such as oral candidiasis.

II. DRUG CALCULATIONS

A. Percentage strength
   1. Percentage strength is the number of parts of the solute (active ingredient) per 100 parts of solution.
   2. To convert from ratio strength to percentage strength, convert the ratio to a fraction and multiply by 100.

EXAMPLE: What is the percentage strength of a 1:2000 solution?

Change 1:2000 to a fraction: 1/2000
Change this to a percentage by dividing 2000 into 1 and multiply the quotient by 100.

$$1 \div 2000 \times 100 = 0.05\%$$

EXAMPLE: What is the percentage strength of a 1:500 solution?

Change 1:500 to a fraction: 1/500
Change this to a percentage by dividing 500 into 1 and multiplying by 100.

$$1 \div 500 \times 100 = 0.2\%$$

   3. To convert from percentage strength to ratio strength, divide by 100 and convert the resulting fraction to a ratio.

EXAMPLE: What is the ratio strength of a 10% solution?

Change 10% to 10/100 or 10:100.
10:100 is the same as 1:10 (10 goes into 100 ten times)
Therefore, a 10% solution has a **1:10 ratio strength.**

B. Dosage calculations

NOTE: 1 ml of a 1% solution (1:100) = 10 mg of solute. (This is a standard rule.)

EXAMPLE: How many milligrams of isoproterenol are in 0.5 ml of a 1:100 solution of the drug?

A 1:100 solution is a 1% solution (1 divided by 100 **x** 100).
1 ml of a 1% solution = 10 mg (the standard rule).
0.5 ml of a 1% solution = 5 mg.

EXAMPLE: How many milligrams of metaproterenol are in 0.2 ml of a 5% solution?

Always go back to the **standard rule: 1 ml of 1% = 10 mg.**
1 ml of a 1% solution = 10 mg.
1 ml of a **5%** solution = 50 mg.
0.2 ml of 50 mg = **10 mg** (0.2 **x** 50 mg).

C. **Calculating children's dosages**
  1. **Young's rule** — uses child's age for 2- to 12-year-old children

$$\frac{\text{age of child}}{\text{age of child} + 12} \times \text{adult dose} = \text{child's dose}$$

  2. **Clark's rule** — uses the weight of the child

$$\frac{\text{weight of child (lb)}}{150} \times \text{adult dose} = \text{child's dose}$$

NOTE: **150 represents the average adult weight in pounds.**

REFERENCES

Eubanks D, Bone R. *Comprehensive Respiratory Care.* 2nd ed. St. Louis: CV Mosby; 1990.
Oakes D. *Clinical Practitioner's Pocket Guide to Respiratory Care.* Old Town, MN: Health Educator Publications; 1984.

PRETEST ANSWERS

1. C

2. C

3. A

4. D

5. D

Pulmonary Function Testing

PRETEST QUESTIONS*

1. Which of the following would best determine the diagnosis of asthma versus emphysema?

A. pre- and post bronchodilator study
B. oxygen saturation monitoring
C. sputum culture
D. complete blood count

2. Reversibility of obstructed airways and improved flowrates following a before-and-after bronchodilator study is considered significant at what percent improvement?

A. 5%
B. 10%
C. 15%
D. 25%

3. Below are the results of a patient's spirometry test before and after bronchodilator therapy.

	Before	After
FEV_1	28% of predicted	61% of predicted
FVC	46% of predicted	82% of predicted
FEV_1/FVC	48%	68%

Which of the following is the correct interpretation of these results?

A. severe restrictive disease, no significant bronchodilator response
B. mild obstructive disease, no significant bronchodilator response
C. severe obstructive disease, significant bronchodilator response
D. mild restrictive disease, significant bronchodilator response

*See answers at the end of the chapter

CHAPTER **12**

Pulmonary Function Testing

I. LUNG VOLUMES AND CAPACITIES

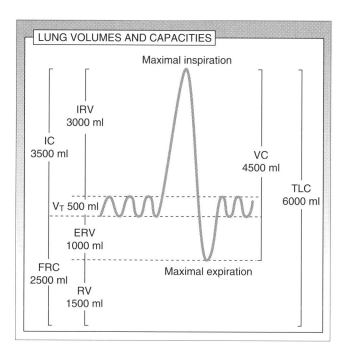

LUNG VOLUMES AND CAPACITIES

A. **Lung volumes**

1. **Tidal volume (V_T)**

   a. The volume of air (usually in milliliters) inhaled or exhaled during a normal breath

   b. Exhaled tidal volume is usually measured with a respirometer or by spirometry.

   c. Decreased or normal with restrictive disease and increased or normal with obstructive disease

   d. Normal value — 500 ml (3 ml/lb of body weight)

2. **Residual volume (RV)**

   a. The volume of air remaining in the lungs following a maximal expiration

   b. Measured most accurately by the helium dilution test

   c. Measured indirectly by RV = FRC − ERV (expiratory reserve volume)

   d. Increased in obstructive disease and decreased in restrictive disease

   e. Normal value — 1200 ml

3. **Inspiratory reserve volume (IRV)**

   a. The maximum volume of air that can be inspired following a normal inspiration

   b. Normally not measured during simple spirometry; should be measured from a slow vital capacity if measurement is needed

   c. May be normal in both obstructive and restrictive disease; therefore, not often clinically significant

   d. Normal value — 3000 ml

4. **Expiratory reserve volume (ERV)**

   a. The volume of air exhaled following a normal expiration

   b. Measured directly by spirometry from a slow vital capacity (VC − IC)

    c. May be normal or decreased in obstructive or restrictive disease

    d. Normal value — 1000 ml (20% to 25% of vital capacity)

B. Lung capacities

   1. Functional residual capacity (FRC)

    a. The amount of air left in the lungs following a normal expiration (ERV + RV)

    b. Measured by the helium dilution test, nitrogen washout test, or body plethysmography

    c. Increased in obstructive disease and decreased in restrictive disease

    d. Normal value — 2400 ml

   2. Inspiratory capacity (IC)

    a. The maximum amount of air that can be inspired following a normal expiration (V_T + IRV)

    b. Measured by simple spirometry from a slow vital capacity

    c. Usually decreased or normal in obstructive or restrictive disease

    d. Normal value — 3000 to 4000 ml (75% to 85% of vital capacity)

   3. Slow vital capacity (SVC) or vital capacity (VC)

    a. The maximum amount of air that can be exhaled following a maximum inspiration (V_T + IRV + ERV)

    b. Measured by simple spirometry

    c. Decreased in restrictive disease and normal or decreased in obstructive disease

    d. Normal value — 4800 ml

NOTE: A decreased vital capacity may be the result of pneumonia, atelectasis, pulmonary edema, or lung cancer.

   4. Forced vital capacity (FVC)

    a. The maximum amount of air that can be exhaled as **fast and forcefully as possible** following a maximum inspiration

    b. Measured by simple spirometry

    c. Used to measure forced expiratory volumes and flows

    d. Decreased in both obstructive and restrictive disease

    e. Normal value — 4800 ml

   5. Total lung capacity (TLC)

    a. The amount of air remaining in the lungs at the end of a maximal inspiration

    b. Calculated by a combination of other measured volumes (FRC + IC or VC + RV)

    c. Decreased in restrictive disease and increased in obstructive disease

    d. Normal value — 6000 ml

NOTE: Total lung capacity will decrease as a result of atelectasis, pulmonary edema, and consolidation and increase in emphysema.

   6. Residual volume:Total lung capacity ratio (RV/TLC)

    a. Percentage of TLC remaining in the lungs after a maximal expiration

    b. Measured by dividing the RV by the TLC and multiplying by 100 to obtain a percentage

    c. Decreased in restrictive disease and increased in obstructive disease

    d. Normal value — 20% to 35%

II. LUNG STUDIES

A. Ventilation studies

   1. Tidal volume (mentioned earlier)

   2. Respiratory rate

    a. The number of breaths in 1 minute

    b. Measured by counting chest excursions for 1 minute

    c. Increased due to hypoxia and hypercapnia and decreased with central respiratory center depression or depression of hypoxic drive in a COPD patient.

    d. Normal value — 10 to 20/min

   3. Minute volume (MV, VE)

    a. The total volume of air inhaled or exhaled in 1 minute. **Calculated by multiplying the respiratory rate by the tidal volume.**

    b. Measured by simple spirometry or at bedside with a respirometer

    c. Increased due to hypoxia, hypercapnia, acidosis, or decreased lung compliance. Decreased due to hyperoxia, hypocapnia, alkalosis, or increased lung compliance.

    d. Normal value — 5 to 10 L/min

B. Flow studies

   1. Forced expiratory volume ($FEV_{0.5}$, FEV_1, FEV_3)

    a. The volume of air exhaled over a specific time interval during the FVC maneuver

    b. Measured over 0.5, 1, or 3 seconds. FEV_1 is the most common measurement.

    c. The severity of airway obstruction may be determined by FEV because it is a measurement at specified time intervals. **FEV is usually decreased in both obstructive and restrictive disease.**

NOTE: FEV may be decreased in restrictive disease because the FVC is below normal and the measurement of FEV is dependent on the FVC. (A better indicator of an obstructive or restrictive disorder is determined from the FEV/FVC ratio.)

2. FEV/FVC ratio
   a. The FEV expressed as a percentage of the FVC
   b. Normal values
      (1) 50% to 60% of the FVC is exhaled in 0.5 second.
      (2) 75% to 85% of the FVC is exhaled in 1 second.
      (3) 94% of the FVC is exhaled in 2 seconds.
      (4) 97% of the FVC is exhaled in 3 seconds.
   c. Obstructive disease is indicated by below-normal values in the FEV/FVC. Patients with restrictive disease have normal or above-normal values.
   d. Because FEV_1 is most commonly measured, look for an FEV_1/FVC of less than 75% to indicate an obstructive disease.

3. Forced expiratory flow ($FEF_{200-1200}$)
   a. The average flowrate of the exhaled air after the first 200 ml during an FVC maneuver
   b. Measured on the spirograph tracing between the 200-ml mark and the 1200-ml mark to determine the average flowrate from the FVC
   c. Decreased in obstructive disease
   d. Normal value — 6 to 7 L/sec (400 L/min)

4. Forced expiratory flow ($FEF_{25\%-75\%}$)
   a. The average flowrate during the middle portion of the FEV
   b. The 25% and 75% points are marked on the spirographic curve from the FVC.
   c. Decreased in obstructive disease
   d. Normal value — 4 to 5 L/sec (250 L/min)

5. Peak flow
   a. The maximum flowrate achieved during an FVC measurement
   b. Measured from an FVC or by a peak flowmeter. (**This is a good bedside test to determine effectiveness of bronchodilator therapy.**)
   c. Decreased in obstructive disease
   d. Normal value — >10 L/sec (600 L/min)

6. Maximum voluntary ventilation (MVV)
   a. The maximum volume of air moved into and out of the lungs voluntarily in 10, 12, or 15 seconds
   b. Tests for overall lung function and ventilatory reserve capacity and identifies air trapping
   c. Decreased in obstructive disease and decreased or normal in restrictive disease
   d. Normal value — 170 L/min

III. OBSTRUCTIVE VERSUS RESTRICTIVE DISEASES

A. Obstructive diseases
   1. Emphysema
   2. Asthma
   3. Chronic bronchitis
   4. Cystic fibrosis
   5. Bronchiectasis

NOTE: These diseases result in *decreased flow studies* (FEV_1, $FEF_{25\%-75\%}$, $FEF_{200-1200}$).

B. Restrictive diseases or disorders
   1. Fibrotic disease
   2. Chest wall disease
   3. Pneumonia
   4. Neuromuscular disease
   5. Pleural disease
   6. Postsurgical patients

NOTE: These diseases result in *decreased volumes* (FRC, FVC, IC, IRV).

C. Severity of disease (by pulmonary function test [PFT] interpretation)
   1. Normal PFT — 80% to 100% of predicted value
   2. Mild disorder — 60% to 79% of predicted value
   3. Moderate disorder — 40% to 59% of predicted value
   4. Severe disorder — <40% of predicted value
D. Predicted values are determined from:
   1. Age
   2. Sex
   3. Height
   4. Ideal body weight
   5. Race

IV. MISCELLANEOUS PULMONARY FUNCTION STUDIES

A. **Before-and-after bronchodilator studies**
1. Used to determine the reversibility of lung dysfunction
2. Asthmatics may be given their routine medication between tests to determine drug effectiveness.
3. Reversibility of obstructed airways and improved flowrates is considered significant for **increases in flow studies of at least 15%.**

B. **Methacholine challenge test**
1. Determines the degree of airway reactivity to methacholine, a drug that stimulates bronchoconstriction
2. May be performed in a before-and-after bronchodilator study or prior to exercise-induced asthma studies
3. Test objective is to determine the minimum level of methacholine that elicits a **20% decrease in FEV$_1$**
4. A physician, bronchodilators, and resuscitation equipment should be present during testing.

V. INTERPRETATION CHART SUMMARY

Pulmonary Function Tests	*Test Results With Obstructive Disease*	*Test Results With Restrictive Disease*
FVC	Decreased	Decreased
IC	Decreased or normal	Decreased
ERV	Decreased or normal	Decreased
V$_T$	Increased	Decreased or normal
FRC	Increased	Decreased
RV	Increased	Decreased
RV/TLC	Increased	Decreased
FEV$_1$	Decreased	Normal (FEV$_1$/FVC)
FEF$_{200-1200}$	Decreased	Normal
FEF$_{25\%-75\%}$	Decreased	Normal
FEV/FVC	Decreased	Normal
MVV	Decreased	Decreased

VI. FLOW-SENSING DEVICE

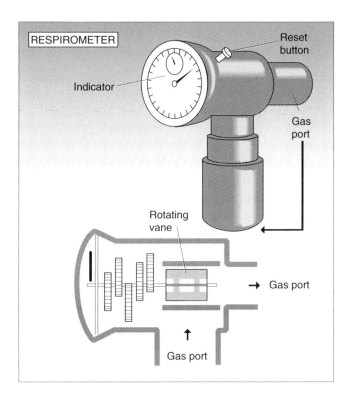

A. **Wright respirometer**
1. A hand-held device frequently used at the patient's bedside to measure vital capacity, tidal volume, and minute volume
2. As the patient's exhaled gas flows through the respirometer, vanes rotate within the device. Through a gear mechanism, the movement of the vanes is indicated on a dial calibrated in liters.
3. This device may also be placed in-line with ventilator circuits to measure the patient's exhaled volume. When used for this purpose, it should be placed on the expiratory side of the circuit as close to the patient as possible.

REFERENCES

Eubanks D, Bone R. *Comprehensive Respiratory Care.* 2nd ed. St. Louis: CV Mosby; 1990.

Ruppell G. *Manual of Pulmonary Function Testing.* 4th ed. St. Louis: CV Mosby; 1986.

Scanlan C, Spearman C. *Egan's Fundamentals of Respiratory Care.* 5th ed. St. Louis: CV Mosby; 1990.

PRETEST ANSWERS

1. A

2. C

3. C

Workbook

CHAPTER 13

▼▼ Pulmonary Patient Assessment

I. PATIENT HISTORY

A. What information should be especially noted when taking a patient history?

B. What does the term "symptomatology" mean?

II. ASSESSMENT OF SYMPTOMS

A. List four common symptoms with which pulmonary patients frequently present.

1.

2.

3.

4.

B. Describe what the following colors of sputum may indicate about a patient's illness.

    1. White and translucent —

    2. Yellow (purulent) —

    3. Green —

    4. Green and foul smelling —

    5. Brown —

    6. Red —

C. Define the term "orthopnea."

D. Define the condition known as paroxysmal nocturnal dyspnea.

E. What is hemoptysis and with which disorders may it be observed?

F. List five sources from which chest pain may originate.

    1.

    2.

3.

4.

5.

III. OTHER PHYSICAL ASSESSMENTS

A. Give a brief description of the following breathing patterns and a condition with which the pattern may be observed.

1. Eupnea —

2. Bradypnea —

3. Apnea —

4. Tachypnea —

5. Hypopnea —

6. Hyperpnea —

7. Kussmaul's respiration —

8. Biot's respiration —

9. Cheyne-Stokes respiration—

B. What may asymmetrical chest movement indicate?

C. What is a "barrel chest" indicative of?

D. What is paradoxical respiration and with what condition may it be observed?

E. Give four examples of muscles that are referred to as accessory muscles of ventilation.

F. What is digital clubbing and when is it observed?

G. Explain what pedal edema is and what causes it.

H. Explain why anemic patients will not necessarily be cyanotic even though moderate to severe hypoxia may be present.

I. Define the following chest deformities:

1. Kyphosis —

2. Scoliosis —

3. Kyphoscoliosis —

4. Lordosis —

5. Pectus carinatum —

6. Pectus excavatum —

J. Is kyphoscoliosis an obstructive or restrictive disorder?

K. Why do chronic lung patients use their accessory muscles during normal ventilation?

L. Under what three conditions may tactile fremitus be decreased?

1.

2.

3.

M. A shift of the trachea toward the lung with diminished breath sounds may indicate what?

N. A shift of the trachea away from the lung with diminished breath sounds may indicate what?

O. A dullness on percussion over a specific lung segment may indicate what?

P. Match the breath sound to the appropriate area in which it is heard.

1. Vesicular _____
    a. Between the scapula and over the sternum

2. Bronchial _____
    b. Over the trachea

3. Bronchovesicular _____
    c. Upper part of sternum, trachea, and main-stem bronchi

4. Tracheal _____
    d. Entire chest wall except the supraclavicular area

Q. Give five examples of conditions in which rales may be heard on auscultation.

1.

2.

3.

4.

5.

R. What causes the wheezing sound heard on auscultation of asthmatics?

S. A chest x-ray showing consolidation may be indicative of what condition?

T. At what level on chest x-ray should the tip of the endotracheal tube be placed?

U. If an endotracheal tube is inserted too far, where would the tube most likely rest? How would you know the tube was inserted too far?

V. Define the following terms:

1. Bradycardia —

2. Tachycardia —

W. What term is used to describe an abnormally low blood pressure?

X. What term is used to describe an abnormally high blood pressure?

IV. REVIEWING THE PATIENT CHART

A. List six areas of the chart that should be reviewed after the patient has been admitted.

1.

2.

3.

4.

5.

6.

B. List the normal values for red blood cell count and white blood cell count.

    1. Red blood cell count

    2. White blood cell count

CHAPTER 14

Oxygen and Medical Gas Therapy

I. STORAGE AND CONTROL OF MEDICAL GASES

A. Medical gas cylinders are constructed of what metal?

B. Large cylinders utilize which safety system to prevent improper regulator/cylinder connection?

C. Small cylinders utilize which safety system to prevent improper regulator/cylinder connection?

D. Match the cylinder gas to its appropriate cylinder color recommended by the Compressed Gas Association.

1. Oxygen _____   a. Gray

2. Helium _____   b. Orange

3. Carbon dioxide _____ c. Light blue

4. Nitrous oxide _____   d. Red

5. Cyclopropane _____   e. Brown

6. Ethylene _____   f. Yellow

7. Air _____   g. Green

E. What is the boiling point of oxygen?

F. How can you determine how many stages a reducing valve has?

G. List the appropriate cylinder factors for the following:

1. H cylinder   _____

2. E cylinder   _____

H. An E cylinder contains 1800 psig of oxygen and is running at 6 L/min through a nasal cannula. Calculate how long the cylinder will run until it is empty.*

I. Where is the needle valve located on a noncompensated flowmeter? If a humidifier is attached to the outlet of the flowmeter, will it read higher or lower than what the patient is actually receiving?

J. Where is the needle valve located on a compensated flowmeter? What happens to the float when the flowmeter is plugged into a wall outlet while it is turned off?

K. On what devices is the Diameter Index Safety System used?

_____

*Answer to problem H: 1 hour 24 minutes

L. With a nebulizer attached to the outlet of a Bourdon gauge regulator, will the gauge read accurately or higher or lower than what the patient is actually receiving?

II. OXYGEN THERAPY

A. List three indications for the use of oxygen.

1.

2.

3.

B. List seven signs and symptoms of hypoxemia.

1.

2.

3.

4.

5.

6.

7.

C. List five complications of oxygen therapy.

   1.

   2.

   3.

   4.

   5.

D. In order to avoid knocking out a COPD patient's "hypoxic drive," at what level must the Pa_{O_2} be maintained?

E. List the four types of hypoxia and give an example of each.

   1.

   2.

   3.

   4.

F. A patient on a 60% oxygen mask is ventilating well but has a Pa_{O_2} of 54 mm Hg. What would be the appropriate course of action?

G. What is the normal hemoglobin level?

H. What is the difference between a low-flow and a high-flow oxygen delivery device?

I. Indicate which oxygen delivery devices are considered high-flow and which low-flow.

1. Nasal cannula _____

2. Simple oxygen mask_____

3. Venturi mask _____

4. Aerosol mask _____

5. Nonrebreathing mask _____

6. Partial rebreathing mask _____

J. What three criteria must be met for a low-flow oxygen device to be considered adequate?

1.

2.

3.

K. List the air:oxygen entrainment ratios at the following percentages:

1. 24% _____

5. 40% _____

2. 28% _____

6. 50% _____

3. 30% _____

7. 60% _____

4. 35% _____

8. 100% _____

L. Calculate the total flow from a nebulizer set on 40% and attached to an oxygen flowmeter running at 12 L/min.*

M. How can you ensure that the flow being delivered from a nebulizer is high enough for the patient's inspiratory needs?

N. A nebulizer is set in the 40% dilution mode and connected to an oxygen flowmeter running at 12 L/min. Downstream there is an air bleed-in at 10 L/min. Calculate the F_{IO_2}.†

O. What is the maximum percentage an oxygen tent is capable of delivering?

---

*Answer to problem L: 48 LPM
†Answer to problem N: .365 or 36.5%

III. OXYGEN ANALYZERS

A. Which oxygen analyzer utilizes the Pauling principle in its operation?

B. List three conditions that affect the accuracy of a polarographic oxygen analyzer.

1.

2.

3.

IV. CO-OXIMETRY

A. What is CO-oximetry?

B. List the signs and symptoms of CO poisoning with the following carboxyhemoglobin level concentrations:

1. 0 to 10% —

2. 10 to 20% —

3. 20 to 40% —

4. 40 to 60% —

5. >60% —

CHAPTER 15

Humidity and Aerosol Therapy

I. HUMIDITY THERAPY

A. Define humidity.

B. List two clinical uses of humidity.

1.

2.

C. Fully saturated inspired air at body temperature contains how many milligrams of water per liter of air? How much vapor pressure (mm Hg)?

1. _____ mg/L

2. _____ mm Hg

D. Define absolute humidity.

E. Define relative humidity and give the equation used to calculate it.

F. The amount of moisture in a volume of air at 25°C is 21 mg of water per liter of air. Calculate the relative humidity. (Note: At 25°C the air can hold 23.04 mg of water per liter of air.)*

G. The inspired gas of a patient contains 18 mg of water per liter of air. Calculate the humidity deficit in mg/L and as a percentage.†

H. List three factors that affect the efficiency of humidifiers.

1.

2.

3.

I. Explain the operation of a pass-over humidifier.

J. Explain the operation of a bubble humidifier.

---

*Answer to problem F: 91%
†Answer to problem G: 26 mg/L and 59%

K. Which humidifiers discussed have the potential to deliver inspired gas at 100% body humidity?

L. What body humidity (%) may be achieved with a heat moisture exchanger?

M. Explain how a heat moisture exchanger works.

II. AEROSOL THERAPY

A. Define aerosol.

B. What is the ideal aerosol particle size for delivery to the airway?

C. List six clinical uses of aerosol therapy.

1.

2.

3.

4.

5.

6.

D. List five factors that affect the penetration and deposition of aerosol particles.

1.

2.

3.

4.

5.

E. Explain the operation of a hydrosphere.

F. What type of fluid should be placed into the couplant chamber of the ultrasonic nebulizer?

G. Which control on the ultrasonic nebulizer determines the particle size? Which controls the volume of aerosol output?

H. List six hazards of ultrasonic nebulizer therapy.

1.

2.

3.

4.

5.

6.

I. Why should heated nebulizers be changed every 12 to 24 hours?

J. The pop-off valves on nebulizers are set at what level to release excess pressure?

K. If the capillary tube of the nebulizer becomes clogged, what effect will this have on its operation?

L. Describe the method for instructing a patient on how to properly administer medication with a metered-dose inhaler.

M. What is the benefit of using spacers or holding chambers on metered-dose inhalers?

CHAPTER 16

Equipment Decontamination/ Infection Control

I. BASIC TERMINOLOGY

A. Describe the difference between disinfection and sterilization.

B. What is a spore?

C. What do the terms "bacteriostatic" and "bactericidal" mean?

D. What is a nosocomial infection?

II. CONDITIONS THAT INFLUENCE ANTIMICROBIAL ACTION

A. List seven factors that influence antimicrobial action.

   1.

2.

3.

4.

5.

6.

7.

B. Why is it necessary to wash equipment thoroughly before the decontamination procedure?

III. THREE MAIN CLASSES OF BACTERIA

A. List the three main classes of bacteria.

1.

2.

3.

B. List six examples of bacilli that are frequently responsible for pneumonia and indicate whether they are gram-negative or gram-positive.

1.

2.

3.

4.

5.

6.

IV. STERILIZATION AND DISINFECTION TECHNIQUES

A. List the normal operating settings for the autoclave.

B. Is autoclaving a sterilizing or disinfecting technique?

C. What is the temperature of the water bath for the pasteurization method of cleaning equipment?

D. Does pasteurization sterilize or disinfect equipment?

E. If equipment to be gas sterilized with ethylene oxide is not thoroughly dried, what may occur?

F. Why is 90% carbon dioxide mixed with the ethylene oxide in the sterilization chamber?

G. List the temperatures and exposure times for warm gas and cold gas sterilization.

    1. Warm gas –

    2. Cold gas —

H. List the two types of glutaraldehyde and their appropriate pH levels.

    1.

    2.

I. List the exposure times needed for a glutaraldehyde solution to be bactericidal and sporicidal.

J. What organism is acetic acid very effective against?

V. IMPORTANT POINTS CONCERNING DECONTAMINATION OF EQUIPMENT

A. What type of solution should be used in reservoirs of nebulizers and humidifiers?

B. Why should equipment be completely dry before being packaged?

VI. ISOLATION PRECAUTIONS

A. A patient is in respiratory isolation. What precautions must be taken to prevent cross-contamination to personnel and visitors?

B. A patient is in strict isolation. What precautions must be taken to prevent cross-contamination to personnel and visitors?

CHAPTER 17

Management of the Airway

I. UPPER AIRWAY OBSTRUCTION

A. List six major causes of upper airway obstruction.

 1.

 2.

 3.

 4.

 5.

 6.

B. List six signs of partial upper airway obstruction.

 1.

 2.

3.

4.

5.

6.

C. List seven signs of complete upper airway obstruction.

1.

2.

3.

4.

5.

6.

7.

D. What are the steps to take in helping a conscious victim with a partial upper airway obstruction?

E. What is the best method of relieving an upper airway obstruction caused by the tongue falling into the back of the throat?

F. What maneuver is used to relieve an upper airway obstruction caused by food or other foreign bodies?

II. ARTIFICIAL AIRWAYS

A. Describe the proper insertion technique for an oropharyngeal airway.

B. List four hazards of the oropharyngeal airway.

1.

2.

3.

4.

C. Why should the oropharyngeal airway never be placed in a conscious patient?

D. Describe the proper insertion technique of the nasopharyngeal airway.

E. What are two hazards of a nasopharyngeal airway?

    1.

    2.

F. List four indications for endotracheal tubes.

    1.

    2.

    3.

    4.

G. List the four normal airway reflexes and what response they elicit when stimulated.

    1.

    2.

    3.

    4.

H. List eight hazards of endotracheal tubes.

    1.

    2.

3.

4.

5.

6.

7.

8.

I. Describe how the MacIntosh and Miller laryngoscope blades are used to visualize the vocal cords.

J. Describe the steps for endotracheal intubation.

K. How far past the vocal cords should the E-T tube be advanced?

L. What is the average distance from the teeth to the carina in the adult?

M. List eight complications of oral E-T tubes.

1.

2.

3.

4.

5.

6.

7.

8.

N. What are McGill forceps used for?

O. List the advantages and complications of nasotracheal tubes.

Advantages:

1.

2.

3.

4.

5.

Complications:

    1.

    2.

    3.

    4.

    5.

P. List five indications for tracheostomy tubes.

    1.

    2.

    3.

    4.

    5.

Q. List the immediate and late complications of tracheostomy tubes.

Immediate:

    1.

    2.

3.

4.

Late:

1.

2.

3.

4.

5.

R. Describe a fenestrated tracheostomy tube and its purpose.

S. Describe the tracheostomy button and its purpose.

T. Describe how speaking tracheostomy tubes work.

III. MAINTENANCE OF ARTIFICIAL AIRWAYS

A. What type of cuff should be utilized on all E-T tubes and tracheostomy tubes?

B. Describe how to inflate a cuff using the minimal leak technique and the minimal occluding volume technique.

C. What is the importance of using the minimal leak or occluding volume technique for cuff inflation?

D. What pressure should the E-T tube cuff be kept below to prevent obstruction of arterial flow, venous flow, and lymphatic flow?

1. Arterial flow —

2. Venous flow —

3. Lymphatic flow —

E. List the steps for endotracheal suctioning.

F. List the suctioning levels for adults, children, and infants.

1. Adults —

2. Children —

3. Infants —

G. Describe how to determine what size suction catheter is appropriate for a given E-T tube size.

H. A patient is intubated with a 6.5-mm E-T tube. What is the appropriate size suction catheter to suction this tube?*

I. List three indications for tracheal suctioning.

   1.

   2.

   3.

J. List five hazards of tracheal suctioning and appropriate techniques to decrease the potential of these hazards.

   1.

   2.

   3.

   4.

   5.

---

*Answer to problem H: 10- to 12-French suction catheter

K. What is a Yankauer suction?

L. What is a coudé suction catheter used for?

IV. ENDOTRACHEAL EXTUBATION

A. Describe the steps in performing E-T tube extubation.

B. List two complications of extubation and appropriate treatment for each.

   1.

   2.

C. What type of oxygen delivery device is most appropriate following extubation and why?

V. LARYNGEAL AND TRACHEAL COMPLICATIONS OF ENDOTRACHEAL TUBES

A. What is the major clinical sign of glottic edema?

B. List four causes of glottic edema.

    1.

    2.

    3.

    4.

C. List three ways of treating glottic edema.

    1.

    2.

    3.

D. Describe subglottic edema.

E. Describe tracheal stenosis and where it is most commonly found in the airway.

F. How may tracheal stenosis at the cuff site be prevented?

VI. CHEST PHYSICAL THERAPY

A. List four chest physical therapy techniques.

1.

2.

3.

4.

B. List four goals of chest physical therapy.

1.

2.

3.

4.

C. List six indications for chest physical therapy.

1.

2.

3.

4.

5.

6.

D. List five contraindications for postural drainage.

1.

2.

3.

4.

5.

E. Describe how you would position a patient to drain the right middle lobe.

F. Describe how you would position a patient to drain the left upper lobe.

G. Describe how you would position a patient to drain the right lower lobe.

H. List five areas over which you should *never* percuss.

1.

2.

3.

4.

5.

I. List seven adverse effects of chest physical therapy.

1.

2.

3.

4.

5.

6.

7.

J. Describe the steps in performing an effective cough maneuver.

CHAPTER 18

Intermittent Positive Pressure Breathing (IPPB) Therapy/Incentive Spirometry

I. INTRODUCTION TO INTERMITTENT POSITIVE PRESSURE BREATHING (IPPB) THERAPY

A. Define intermittent positive pressure breathing.

B. List four factors that make IPPB effective.

1.

2.

3.

4.

II. PHYSIOLOGIC EFFECTS OF IPPB

A. List six physiologic effects of IPPB.

    1.

    2.

    3.

    4.

    5.

    6.

B. Explain how airway resistance and lung compliance affect the delivered tidal volume when using a pressure-limited ventilator for IPPB.

C. The respiratory care practitioner should deliver a tidal volume of _____ ml/kg of body weight during IPPB.

D. List four reasons why IPPB may increase the patient's work of breathing.

    1.

    2.

    3.

4.

E. The patient should not be required to generate more than _____ cm H_2O to cycle the IPPB unit into inspiration.

III. INDICATIONS FOR IPPB THERAPY

A. List seven indications for IPPB therapy.

1.

2.

3.

4.

5.

6.

7.

B. List two conditions that result in an increased airway resistance.

1.

2.

IV. HAZARDS OF IPPB THERAPY

A. List eight hazards of IPPB therapy.

1.

2.

3.

4.

5.

6.

7.

8.

B. What is a common complaint from a patient being excessively ventilated during IPPB?

C. Give a set of arterial blood gas results that would indicate you were knocking out a COPD patient's hypoxic drive during IPPB.

1. pH —

2. Pa_{CO_2} —

3. Pa_{O_2} —

D. Explain how IPPB may cause a decrease in cardiac output.

E. Explain how IPPB may cause an elevation in intracranial pressure (ICP).

F. What is the normal value for ICP?

G. How may the respiratory care practitioner decrease the potential of elevating the ICP during IPPB therapy?

H. In what type of patient is a pneumothorax induced by IPPB most common?

V. CONTRAINDICATIONS FOR IPPB THERAPY

A. List two absolute contraindications of IPPB.

1.

2.

B. List eight relative contraindications of IPPB.

1.

2.

3.

4.

5.

6.

7.

8.

VI. IPPB IN THE TREATMENT OF PULMONARY EDEMA

A. How does IPPB aid in the treatment of pulmonary edema?

B. What measures, other than IPPB, should be employed to treat pulmonary edema?

VII. PROPER ADMINISTRATION OF IPPB

A. List the steps involved in the proper administration of IPPB.

B. If the patient's pulse increases more than _____ beats per minute during IPPB therapy, the treatment should be stopped immediately and the physician notified.

C. Following IPPB therapy, what information should be recorded in the patient's chart?

VIII. CHARACTERISTICS OF SPECIFIC IPPB UNITS

A. When gas enters the Bird Mark 7 unit, what is the first control through which it travels?

B. What determines the degree of sensitivity for the patient to cycle the unit into inspiration on the Bird Mark 7?

C. Describe the flow characteristics at end inspiration with the Bird Mark 7.

D. What liter flow is available on the Bird Mark 7 when air mix is used and when it is not used?

E. How does increasing the flowrate on the Bird Mark 7 affect the inspiratory time?

F. What kind of flow-wave form occurs when the Bird Mark 7 is set on 100% and on air mix?

   1. 100% —

2. Air mix —

G. What ends inspiration on the Bird Mark 7?

H. What ends inspiration on the Bennett PR-2?

I. What is the terminal flow control used for on the Bennett PR-2?

J. What is the effect on F_{IO_2} when the terminal flow control is used on the Bennett PR-2?

IX. IMPORTANT FACTORS TO CONSIDER WHEN VENTILATING A PATIENT WITH A PRESSURE-LIMITED IPPB MACHINE

A. What effect do the following conditions have on the delivered tidal volume (increase or decrease)?

1. Increased airway resistance —

2. Decreased airway resistance —

3. Increased lung compliance —

4. Decreased lung compliance —

5. Increased peak pressure —

6. Decreased peak pressure —

7. Increased flowrate —

8. Decreased flowrate —

B. What effect do the following conditions have on the inspiratory time (increase or decrease)?

1. Increased airway resistance —

2. Decreased airway resistance —

3. Increased lung compliance —

4. Decreased lung compliance —

5. Increased flowrate —

6. Decreased flowrate —

X. PROBLEMS ENCOUNTERED IN ADMINISTERING IPPB AND CORRECTIVE ACTIONS

A. List six corrective actions to take if the patient is having difficulty cycling the IPPB machine off.

1.

2.

3.

4.

5.

6.

B. If the patient complains of tingling in the fingers or dizziness during an IPPB treatment, what corrective action should be taken?

C. List five corrective actions to take if nebulization of medications is not occurring?

1.

2.

3.

4.

5.

D. You notice during inspiration that the manometer needle remains in the negative area for half of inspiration before moving to the positive area during the last half of inspiration. What machine adjustment would correct this?

E. While the patient is exhaling, the IPPB machine cycles into inspiration. How may this be corrected?

XI. INCENTIVE SPIROMETRY (SUSTAINED MAXIMAL INSPIRATORY THERAPY)

A. List six goals of incentive spirometry.

1.

2.

3.

4.

5.

6.

B. List two guidelines for effective incentive spirometry.

1.

2.

C. List *four hazards* of incentive spirometry.

1.

2.

3.

4.

D. Describe the ideal inspiratory pattern for effective incentive spirometry.

CHAPTER **19**

Cardiopulmonary
Resuscitation/Manual
Resuscitators

I. CARDIOPULMONARY RESUSCITATION (CPR) TECHNIQUES

A. What technique is preferred to open the airway of an unconscious victim?

B. What technique is used to expel a foreign body from a victim's airway?

C. What is the appropriate action to take when the victim has been determined to be breathless?

D. What is the compression-to-breath rate for one-rescuer CPR on an adult victim? Two-rescuer CPR?

    1. One rescuer — _____ compressions, _____ breaths

    2. Two rescuers — _____ compressions, _____ breaths

E. What artery is palpated in the adult to determine the presence or absence of a pulse?

II. ADULT, CHILD, AND INFANT CPR MODIFICATIONS

A. What is the compression-to-breath rate for the child and infant during one-rescuer CPR?

    1. Child — _____ compressions, _____ breaths

    2. Infant — _____ compressions, _____ breaths

B. If the victim has a pulse but is not breathing, at what rate should you ventilate the following victims?

    1. Adult —

    2. Child —

    3. Infant —

C. List the appropriate depth for chest compressions on the following victims:

    1. Adult —

    2. Child —

    3. Infant —

III. CPR — SPECIAL CONSIDERATIONS

A. Compressions achieve only _____ % to _____ % of normal blood flow.

B. What is the best indication of adequate cerebral blood flow during CPR?

C. List three hazards of CPR.

1.

2.

3.

IV. MANUAL RESUSCITATORS

A. List three uses of manual resuscitators.

1.

2.

3.

B. Why is it important to use a reservoir attachment on a manual resuscitator?

C. List four criteria that will aid in delivery of the highest oxygen percentage to the patient.

1.

2.

3.

4.

D. List three hazards of manual resuscitators.

1.

2.

3.

E. Describe mouth-to-valve mask ventilation.

CHAPTER **20**

Arterial Blood Gas Interpretation

I. ARTERIAL BLOOD GAS (ABG) ANALYSIS

A. What blood gas value is used to determine the following:

1. Alveolar ventilation —

2. Arterial oxygenation —

3. Oxygen delivery to the tissues —

4. Acid-base status of the blood —

B. Where and by what method is mixed venous blood obtained?

C. Describe how to perform the modified Allen's test. Why is it performed?

205

D. Describe the steps taken to obtain an arterial blood gas sample from the radial artery.

II. ARTERIAL OXYGENATION

A. What is the Pa_{O_2} a measurement of?

B. For every 1 mm Hg of Pa_{O_2} there is/are _____ ml of oxygen dissolved in the plasma.

C. Write the equation used to calculate alveolar oxygen tension.

D. Given the following data, calculate the patient's P(A–a) gradient.*

pH — 7.35
Pa_{CO_2} — 44 torr
HCO_3 — 26 mEq/L
Pa_{O_2} — 135 torr
F_{IO_2} — 1.0
Barometric pressure — 747 torr

E. Define P(A–a) gradient.

_____

*Answer to problem D: 510 mm Hg

F. If the oxyhemoglobin dissociation curve is shifted to the right, what is the effect on hemoglobin's affinity for oxygen?

G. What conditions will shift the curve to the right?

H. If the oxyhemoglobin dissociation curve is shifted to the left, what is the effect on hemoglobin's affinity for oxygen?

I. What conditions will shift the curve to the left?

J. Explain the Haldane effect.

K. Explain the Bohr effect.

L. List the normal Pa_{O_2} levels according to age.

Age	Pa_{O_2} (mm Hg)
<60	
60	
65	
70	
75	
80	

M. Define the levels of hypoxemia.

60 to 79 mm Hg _____

40 to 59 mm Hg _____

<40 mm Hg _____

N. What is the normal value for arterial oxygen saturation (SaO_2)?

III. CARBON DIOXIDE TRANSPORT AND ALVEOLAR VENTILATION

A. By what mechanism does carbon dioxide enter the blood?

B. What percentage of the atmosphere is composed of carbon dioxide?

C. List three ways that carbon dioxide is carried in the blood.

1.

2.

3.

D. What is the normal Pa_{CO_2} level?

E. What effect does hyperventilation have on Pa_{CO_2}?

F. What effect does hypoventilation have on Pa_{CO_2}?

G. Define the following terms:

1. Hypocapnia —

2. Hypercapnia —

H. What three mechanisms affect Pa_{CO_2}?

1.

2.

3.

IV. ACID-BASE BALANCE (pH)

A. Write the Henderson-Hasselbalch equation.

B. Using the Henderson-Hasselbalch equation, determine the following:

1. If base (HCO_3) decreases and acid (Pa_{CO_2}) remains the same, the pH will_____ .

2. If base (HCO_3) increases and acid (Pa_{CO_2}) remains the same, the pH will _____ .

3. If acid (Pa_{CO_2}) increases and base (HCO_3) remains the same, the pH will _____ .

4. If acid (Pa_{CO_2}) decreases and base (HCO_3) remains the same, the pH will_____ .

C. The ratio of HCO_3 to H_2CO_3 is _____ when the pH is 7.40.

D. What is the normal value for arterial blood pH?

E. Define acidemia.

F. Define alkalemia.

G. A review of blood gas results shows that an acidemia is present. Write examples of a respiratory acidemia and a metabolic acidemia.

H. What is the normal value for HCO_3 levels in arterial blood?

I. What does the term "compensation" refer to in ABG interpretation?

V. ARTERIAL BLOOD GAS INTERPRETATION

A. List the normal arterial blood gas values for neonates.

pH

Pa_{CO_2}

Pa_{O_2}

HCO_3

B. List the normal capillary blood gas values for neonates.

pH

P_{CO_2}

Pa_{O_2}

HCO_3

B.E.

NOTE: Answers to the practice ABG problems are at the end of this chapter.

C. pH —7.21

Pa$_{CO_2}$ — 66 mm Hg

HCO$_3$ — 24 mEq/L

Pa$_{O_2}$ — 68 mm Hg

B.E. — 0

1. Acid-base status:

2. Ventilatory status:

3. Metabolic status:

4. Oxygenation status:

5. Interpretation:

6. Corrective measure(s):

D. pH — 7.55

Pa$_{CO_2}$ — 24 mm Hg

HCO$_3$ — 23 mEq/L

Pa$_{O_2}$ — 94 mm Hg

B.E. — –1

1. Acid-base status:

2. Ventilatory status:

3. Metabolic status:

    4. Oxygenation status:

    5. Interpretation:

    6. Corrective measure(s):

E. pH — 7.24
   Pa_{CO_2} — 41 mm Hg
   HCO_3 — 16 mEq/L
   Pa_{O_2} — 86 mm Hg
   B.E. — –8

    1. Acid-base status:

    2. Ventilatory status:

    3. Metabolic status:

    4. Oxygenation status:

    5. Interpretation:

    6. Corrective measure(s):

F. pH — 7.42

Pa$_{CO_2}$ — 43 mm Hg

HCO$_3$ — 25 mEq/L

Pa$_{O_2}$ — 51 mm Hg

B.E. — +1

1. Acid-base status:

2. Ventilatory status:

3. Metabolic status:

4. Oxygenation status:

5. Interpretation:

6. Corrective measure(s):

G. pH — 7.36

Pa$_{CO_2}$ — 62 mm Hg

HCO$_3$ — 36 mEq/L

Pa$_{O_2}$ — 58 mm Hg

B.E. — +12

1. Acid-base status:

2. Ventilatory status:

3. Metabolic status:

4. Oxygenation status:

5. Interpretation:

6. Corrective measure(s):

H. pH — 7.19

Pa_{CO_2} — 23 mm Hg

HCO_3 — 11 mEq/L

Pa_{O_2} — 88 mm Hg

B.E. — −13

1. Acid-base status:

2. Ventilatory status:

3. Metabolic status:

4. Oxygenation status:

5. Interpretation:

6. Corrective measure(s):

VI. BLOOD GAS ANALYZERS

A. Identify what each blood gas electrode measures:

1. Sanz electrode —

2. Severinghaus electrode —

3. Clark electrode —

VII. OXYGEN SATURATION MONITORING (PULSE OXIMETRY)

A. On what principle is the measurement of Sa_{O_2} by pulse oximeter based?

B. What is the advantage of pulse oximetry?

C. List the disadvantages of pulse oximeters.

VIII. TRANSCUTANEOUS MONITORING OF Pa_{CO_2} AND Pa_{O_2}

A. On what type of patient is transcutaneous monitoring most commonly utilized?

B. What is the purpose of heating the probe that is attached to the skin?

C. What is the advantage of transcutaneous monitoring?

D. List the disadvantages of transcutaneous monitoring.

E. What is the normal Pa_{O_2} in the neonate?

ARTERIAL BLOOD GAS INTERPRETATION

Answer to problem C:

1. Acid-base status: Acidemia
2. Ventilatory status: Increased Pa_{CO_2} — hypoventilation resulting in decreased pH level
3. Metabolic status: Normal HCO_3
4. Oxygenation status: Decreased Pa_{O_2} (mild hypoxemia)
5. Interpretation: Uncompensated (acute) respiratory acidemia. It is uncompensated because the HCO_3 level is still within normal limits.
6. Corrective measure(s): Intubate and place on mechanical ventilator. If already on ventilator, increase the tidal volume or rate to increase the patient's minute ventilation. This will result in a decrease in the Pa_{CO_2}.

Answer to problem D:

1. Acid-base status: Alkalemia
2. Ventilatory status: Decreased Pa_{CO_2} — hyperventilation
3. Metabolic status: Normal HCO_3
4. Oxygenation status: Normal Pa_{O_2}
5. Interpretation: Uncompensated (acute) respiratory alkalemia (hyperventilation). It is uncompensated because the HCO_3 level is still within normal limits.
6. Corrective measure(s): If ventilator-induced, decrease the tidal volume and respiratory rate or add mechanical dead space. If patient is not on ventilator, eliminate the stimulus causing the hyperventilation, such as anxiety, pain, fever, etc.

NOTE: **If this blood gas indicated hypoxemia with hyperventilation, increasing the FIO_2 would be the appropriate corrective measure.**

Answer to problem E:

1. Acid-base status: Acidemia
2. Ventilatory status: Normal Pa_{CO_2}
3. Metabolic status: Decreased HCO_3 level resulting in decreased pH level.
4. Oxygenation status: Normal Pa_{O_2}
5. Interpretation: Uncompensated (acute) metabolic acidemia. It is uncompensated because the Pa_{CO_2} is still within normal limits.
6. Corrective measure(s): Administer sodium bicarbonate ($NaHCO_3$) — no ventilator or oxygen concentration changes are necessary.

Answer to problem F:

1. Acid-base status: Normal pH
2. Ventilatory status: Normal Pa_{CO_2}
3. Metabolic status: Normal HCO_3
4. Oxygenation status: Decreased Pa_{O_2} (moderate hypoxemia)
5. Interpretation: Normal acid-base status with moderate hypoxemia
6. Corrective measure(s): Increase the F_{IO_2} unless the patient is already on an O_2 mask at 60% or greater, then place on CPAP. If the patient is on a ventilator, PEEP should be applied or increased if on 60% oxygen or higher. If on less than 60%, increase the F_{IO_2}.

Answer to problem G:

1. Acid-base status: Normal pH
2. Ventilatory status: Increased Pa_{CO_2} — hypoventilation resulting in acidemia
3. Metabolic status: Increased HCO_3 level compensating for initial acidemia.
4. Oxygenation status: Decreased Pa_{O_2} (moderate hypoxemia)
5. Interpretation: Compensated (chronic) respiratory acidemia. These blood gases are typical of the severe COPD patient with chronic hypercapnia and hypoxemia. The pH was initially decreased due to the increased Pa_{CO_2} levels. The HCO_3 then increased to return the acidotic pH back to the normal range. Thus, this is considered a compensated respiratory acidemia.
6. Corrective measure(s): Since these gases are considered normal for the severe COPD patient, no changes are necessary.

Answer to problem H:

1. Acid-base status: Acidemia
2. Ventilatory status: Decreased Pa_{CO_2} (hyperventilation)
3. Metabolic status: Decreased HCO_3 level resulting in acidemia
4. Oxygenation status: Normal Pa_{O_2}
5. Interpretation: Partially compensated metabolic acidemia. The decreased HCO_3 level resulted in the acidemia. The lungs have begun compensating by hyperventilation, thus increasing the pH. Since the pH level has not yet reached normal levels, it is considered to be only *partially* compensated.
6. Corrective measure(s): Administer $NaHCO_3$. No respiratory parameter changes are necessary. As the pH begins to increase after the $NaHCO_3$ administration, the Pa_{CO_2} should begin to increase as the stimulus to hyperventilate lessens.

CHAPTER 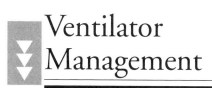21

Ventilator Management

I. NEGATIVE- VERSUS POSITIVE-PRESSURE VENTILATORS

A. List two types of negative-pressure ventilators and give the advantages and disadvantages of each.

    1.

    2.

B. List the two types of positive-pressure ventilators.

    1.

    2.

C. What type of ventilator is utilized on neonates? What effect do lung compliance and airway resistance have on delivered tidal volumes?

II. VENTILATOR CONTROLS

A. Describe the following modes of ventilation:

   1. Control mode —

   2. Assist mode —

   3. Assist-control mode —

B. At what level should the sensitivity be set on the ventilator for the patient to cycle it into inspiration?

C. Describe synchronized intermittent mandatory ventilation (SIMV).

D. Describe pressure support ventilation (PSV).

E. Describe continuous positive airway pressure (CPAP).

F. List six indications for continuous positive airway pressure (CPAP).

   1.

   2.

3.

4.

5.

6.

G. List four complications of CPAP.

1.

2.

3.

4.

H. As the oxygenation status of a patient on a mask worsens, at what point should CPAP be employed?

I. How do you determine what initial tidal volume setting should be used on a ventilator patient?

J. Describe bilevel positive airway pressure (BiPAP).

K. What is minute ventilation (volume) and how is it determined?

L. Calculate the ventilator tubing compliance when the volume is set at 300 ml (0.3L) and generating a pressure in the tubing of 60 cm H_2O.*

M. Using the tubing compliance in part (L), calculate the corrected tidal volume when the patient is on 800 ml tidal volume and has a peak inspiratory pressure of 28 cm H_2O.†

N. How is anatomic dead space calculated?

O. List the potential sources of leaks on the ventilator that will affect delivered tidal volume.

P. If the spirometer bellows on the MA-1 ventilator rises during inspiration, what is most likely the problem?

Q. On initial ventilator setup, the respiratory rate should be set within what range?

R. Explain the effect inspiratory flowrate has on inspiratory time.

---

*$300 \div 60 = 5$ ml/cm H_2O
†$28 \times 5 = 140$; $800 - 140 = 660$ ml

S. What is the normal I:E ratio for adults and infants? Write the equation for calculating I:E ratio.

1. Adults —

2. Infants —

3. I:E ratio =

T. List the three ventilator controls that alter the I:E ratio and what effect they have on inspiratory and expiratory time when they are increased or decreased.

U. A patient has been set up with an inverse I:E ratio. How would you adjust the flowrate (increase or decrease) to place the patient on a 1:2 I:E ratio?

V. List seven conditions that may cause the high-pressure alarm on the ventilator to be activated.

1.

2.

3.

4.

5.

6.

7.

W. What is the proper method for setting sigh volume?

X. Describe positive end-expiratory pressure (PEEP).

Y. List the indications for PEEP.

Z. List the hazards of PEEP.

AA. What is optimal PEEP?

BB. If the mixed venous P_{O_2} ($P\overline{v}_{O_2}$) drops below _____ mm Hg after the initiation of PEEP, this would indicate a drop in cardiac output and reduced oxygen delivery to the tissues.

III. INDICATIONS FOR MECHANICAL VENTILATION

A. List four indications for mechanical ventilation.

1.

2.

3.

4.

B. A Pa_{CO_2} of greater than _____ mm Hg indicates ventilatory failure and a need for mechanical ventilator assistance.

IV. COMMON CRITERIA FOR INITIATION OF MECHANICAL VENTILATION

A. List six criteria indicating that mechanical ventilatory assistance is necessary.

1.

2.

3.

4.

5.

6.

B. What is a normal dead space:tidal volume ratio?

C. What does an inadequate negative inspiratory force indicate physiologically?

V. GOALS OF MECHANICAL VENTILATION

A. List five goals of mechanical ventilation.

1.

2.

3.

4.

5.

B. How does mechanical ventilation increase alveolar ventilation?

VI. COMPLICATIONS OF MECHANICAL VENTILATION

A. List eight complications of mechanical ventilation.

1.

2.

3.

4.

5.

6.

7.

8.

B. What causes mechanical ventilator patients to be more prone to respiratory infections?

C. What are the two causes of decreased urinary output for mechanical ventilator patients?

D. What effects can malnutrition have on ventilator patients?

VII. DEAD SPACE

A. Define the three types of dead space.

1.

2.

3.

B. A tracheostomy reduces the amount of dead space by _____ %.

C. What is the purpose of adding mechanical dead space to the ventilator circuit?

D. Mechanical dead space should be added *only* to patients in which ventilator modes?

E. A 150-lb (68 kg) male patient is breathing 10 times per minute with an average tidal volume of 450 ml. Calculate this patient's alveolar ventilation.[*]

VIII. LUNG COMPLIANCE

A. Define compliance.

B. Define dynamic lung compliance and write the equation for calculating it.

C. Define static lung compliance and write the equation for calculating it.

D. Calculate the static lung compliance given the following data.[†]

V$_T$ — 750 ml   PEEP — 8 cm H$_2$O

Flowrate — 50 L/min   PIP — 46 cm H$_2$O

                                                           Plateau pressure — 28 cm H$_2$O

---

[*]Answer to Dead Space problem E: 3 LPM $\frac{(450 - 150)}{300}$ x 10 x 10 = 3000 ml or 3 L

[†] $\dfrac{750}{\underset{(20)}{28-8}}$ = 37.5 ml/cm H$_2$O

E. What does a decreasing static lung compliance indicate about the patient's pulmonary status?

F. List eight conditions that would lead to a decreased static lung compliance.

1.

2.

3.

4.

5.

6.

7.

8.

G. What is a normal static lung compliance for a ventilator patient?

IX. VENTILATION OF THE HEAD TRAUMA PATIENT

A. How should the flowrate be altered on a head trauma patient and why?

B. What should the Pa_{CO_2} levels be maintained at for a head trauma patient and why?

X. WEANING FROM MECHANICAL VENTILATION

A. List nine criteria for weaning from mechanical ventilation.

1.

2.

3.

4.

5.

6.

7.

8.

9.

B. Before a patient is extubated, the F_{IO_2} should be _____ or less.

C. List two types of weaning techniques.

1.

2.

XI. PRACTICE VENTILATOR PROBLEMS

NOTE: **Answers to ventilator practice problems at end of chapter.**

A. A 65-kg (143-lb) patient is on an assist-control rate of 10, tidal volume of 1000 ml (1L), and an F_{IO_2} of 0.5. ABG results are as follows:

pH — 7.58

Pa_{CO_2} — 25 torr

P_{O_2} — 99 torr

What is the appropriate recommendation?

a. Increase the respiratory rate.

b. Decrease the tidal volume.

c. Decrease the sensitivity.

d. Increase the F_{IO_2}.

B. A spontaneously breathing 44-year-old patient is on a 60% oxygen mask with the following ABG values:

pH — 7.45

Pa_{CO_2} — 45 torr

Pa_{O_2} — 56 torr

What is the appropriate measure to take?

a. Place on 90% nonrebreather.

b. Place on assist-control ventilation.

c. Place on control ventilation.

d. Place on CPAP.

C. A 36-year-old woman is on the following ventilator settings:

Assist-control rate — 10

Tidal volume — 650 ml (0.65L)

F_{IO_2} — 0.4

The ABG results are:

pH — 7.22

Pa_{CO_2} — 61 torr

Pa_{O_2} — 75 torr

HCO_3 — 26 mEq/L

B.E. — +1

What is the appropriate ventilator change?

a. Decrease rate.

b. Decrease tidal volume.

c. Increase tidal volume.

d. Increase F_{IO_2}.

D. A 65-kg (143-lb) patient is on a ventilator with the following settings:

Control mode

Rate — 6

Tidal volume — 800 ml

F_{IO_2} — 0.4

The ABG results are:

pH — 7.26

Pa_{CO_2} — 59 torr

Pa_{O_2} — 80 torr

HCO_3 — 23 mEq/L

B.E. — −1

What is the appropriate recommendation?

a. Increase rate.

b. Add mechanical deadspace.

c. Decrease tidal volume.

d. Increase F_{IO_2}.

E. A 45-year-old woman with ARDS is being ventilated on the following settings:

Assist-control mode
Rate — 12
Tidal volume — 700 ml
F_{IO_2} — 0.8
PEEP — 10 cm H_2O

The ABG results are:

pH — 7.41
Pa_{CO_2} — 37 torr
Pa_{O_2} — 158 torr

What is the appropriate recommendation?

a. Decrease F_{IO_2}.

b. Decrease PEEP.

c. Decrease tidal volume.

d. Decrease rate.

XII. VENTILATOR FLOW WAVE CAPABILITIES

A. List the four types of flow patterns and describe their characteristics.

1.

2.

3.

4.

B. Which type of flow pattern would benefit a patient with increased airway resistance?

Answer to problem A: b — decrease tidal volume

Answer to problem B: d — place on CPAP

Answer to problem C: c — increase tidal volume

Answer to problem D: a — increase rate

Answer to problem E: a — decrease F_{IO_2}

CHAPTER 22

Lung Disorders

I. CHRONIC OBSTRUCTIVE PULMONARY DISEASE (COPD)

A. What diseases are classified as COPD?

B. Define emphysema.

C. Which type of emphysema is usually associated with alpha$_1$-antitrypsin deficiency?

D. What is a bleb?

E. What causes an emphysema patient to have an increased functional residual capacity (FRC)?

F. Is an emphysema patient's lung compliance normal, increased, or decreased?

G. List nine signs and symptoms of emphysema.

   1.

   2.

   3.

   4.

   5.

   6.

   7.

   8.

   9.

H. What is characteristic about an emphysema patient's chest x-ray?

I. Which pulmonary function values would be decreased for an emphysema patient?

J. Which oxygen delivery device is most acceptable for use on a patient with emphysema who is chronically hypoxemic?

K. What should the Pa_{O_2} be maintained at on a patient with emphysema who is chronically hypoxemic?

L. Define chronic bronchitis.

M. In which type of COPD is there an increase in the size of mucous glands and an increase in the number of goblet cells?

N. Define asthma.

O. Describe the difference between extrinsic and intrinsic asthma.

P. When mast cells in the airway are stimulated, what five substances are released?

1.

2.

3.

4.

5.

Q. The release of the substances in the previous question results in:

1.

2.

3.

4.

5.

R. What does the term "paradoxical pulse" indicate?

S. Write a set of ABG values that would be normal for a severe emphysema patient and one for an asthmatic in mild-to-moderate acute distress.

Emphysema	*Asthmatic*
pH —	pH —
Pa_{CO_2} —	Pa_{CO_2} —
Pa_{O_2} —	Pa_{O_2} —
HCO_3 —	HCO_3 —
B.E. —	B.E. —

T. What type of white blood cell is characteristically elevated in the sputum of an asthmatic?

U. What does cromolyn sodium do and when is it to be administered?

V. What bronchodilator is commonly administered intravenously for the treatment of status asthmaticus?

W. What does the term "status asthmaticus" refer to?

X. List the proper treatment modalities for emphysema.

Y. List the proper treatment modalities for asthma.

Z. Define cystic fibrosis.

AA. What respiratory medication is frequently used to aid in thinning the secretions of a patient with cystic fibrosis?

BB. Define bronchiectasis.

II. LOWER RESPIRATORY TRACT INFECTIONS

A. Define pneumonia.

B. What decreased airway defense mechanisms may lead to the invasion of pathogenic organisms?

C. What causes the consolidation of specific lung areas with pneumonia.

D. List six signs and symptoms of pneumonia.

1.

2.

3.

4.

5.

6.

E. List four types of bacterial pneumonias. Note which type is the most common.

1.

2.

3.

4.

F. List the proper treatment modalities for pneumonia.

G. What medication is commonly used to treat *Pneumocystis carinii* pneumonia?

H. Define lung abscess.

I. What are the most common microorganisms responsible for lung abscesses?

J. List the signs and symptoms of lung abscess.

K. List the treatment modalities for lung abscess.

III. OTHER LUNG DISORDERS

A. Define cardiogenic pulmonary edema.

B. List four causes of cardiogenic pulmonary edema.

1.

2.

3.

4.

C. What are the two forces that maintain fluid in the capillaries?

1.

2.

D. Which one of these forces, when increased, causes pulmonary edema?

E. Define orthopnea.

F. Define paroxysmal nocturnal dyspnea.

G. List the signs and symptoms of pulmonary edema.

H. What chest x-ray findings are characteristic for a patient with pulmonary edema?

I. List the treatment modalities for pulmonary edema.

J. Define pulmonary embolism.

K. List three causes for pulmonary embolism.

    1.

    2.

    3.

L. List the signs and symptoms of pulmonary embolism.

M. List the treatment modalities for pulmonary embolism.

N. Define acute respiratory distress syndrome (ARDS).

O. List the various causes of ARDS.

P. What effect does decreased surfactant production have on the lung compliance of a patient with ARDS?

Q. List the signs and symptoms of ARDS.

R. List the treatment modalities for ARDS.

S. What effect does the lung compliance of a patient with ARDS have on ventilator peak inspiratory pressure?

T. Define pneumothorax.

U. Define tension pneumothorax.

V. List the signs and symptoms of a pneumothorax.

W. What are characteristic features of a pneumothorax on chest x-ray?

X. List the treatment modalities for a pneumothorax.

Y. Define pleural effusion.

Z. List the signs and symptoms of a pleural effusion.

AA. What are characteristic features of a pleural effusion on chest x-ray?

BB. List the treatment modalities for pleural effusion.

IV. SLEEP APNEA

A. Describe obstructive sleep apnea.

B. What is the most effective method for treating obstructive sleep apnea?

C. What is the difference in respiratory effort observed in a patient with obstructive sleep apnea and a patient with central sleep apnea?

D. List five symptoms of obstructive sleep apnea.

1.

2.

3.

4.

5.

E. Describe central sleep apnea.

F. What disorders are associated with obstructive sleep apnea and central sleep apnea?

Obstructive   *Central*

G. List four symptoms of central sleep apnea.

1.

2.

3.

4.

CHAPTER 23

▼▼ Respiratory Medications

I. CLASSIFICATION OF RESPIRATORY MEDICATIONS

A. List four types of diluents and what each is used for.

1.

2.

3.

4.

B. What type of medication is acetylcysteine (Mucomyst) and what is its primary use?

C. List the side effects of acetylcysteine.

D. Identify three receptors that are stimulated by sympathomimetic drugs and give their location and response to stimulation.

1.

2.

3.

E. When is racemic epinephrine most commonly used?

F. Indicate whether the following medications are considered sympathomimetic bronchodilators.

	Yes	*No*
Acetylcysteine	_____	_____
Isoetharine	_____	_____
Atropine	_____	_____
Isoproterenol	_____	_____
Albuterol	_____	_____
Theophylline	_____	_____
Terbutaline	_____	_____

G. Which sympathomimetic bronchodilator is the strongest beta$_2$-receptor stimulator?

H. What classification of bronchodilator is atropine?

I. What other conditions is atropine used for?

J. Give an example of a phosphodiesterase inhibitor.

K. What is the purpose of administering ethanol to a patient with pulmonary edema?

L. List three neuromuscular blocking agents and each one's purpose in respiratory care.

   1.

   2.

   3.

M. Which one of the three neuromuscular blockers releases histamine?

N. The paralyzing effects of nondepolarizing agents may be reversed with the administration of what two drugs?

   1.

   2.

O. List three steroids that are aerosolized to prevent or reduce airway inflammation in asthma or reduce swelling associated with glottic edema.

   1.

   2.

   3.

II. DRUG CALCULATIONS

A. Calculate the percentage strength of a 1:1000 solution.

B. What is the ratio strength of a 20% solution?

C. How many milligrams (mg) of isoproterenol are in 0.25 ml of a 1:100 preparation of the drug?

D. How many milligrams of metaproterenol are in 0.3 ml of a 5% solution of the drug?

E. Write the two equations used to calculate children's medication doses and identify both by name.

   1.

   2.

CHAPTER 24

Pulmonary Function Testing

I. LUNG VOLUMES AND CAPACITIES

A. Define the following volumes and give their normal values:

   1. Tidal volume (V_T) —

   2. Residual volume (RV) —

   3. Inspiratory reserve volume (IRV) —

   4. Expiratory reserve volume (ERV) —

B. Describe the methods used to measure the following volumes and give examples of diseases or conditions that may lead to a decrease or increase in the volume.

   1. Tidal volume —

   2. Residual volume —

   3. Inspiratory reserve volume —

4. Expiratory reserve volume —

C. Define the following capacities and give their normal values:

1. Functional residual capacity (FRC) —

2. Inspiratory capacity (IC) —

3. Vital capacity (VC) —

4. Forced vital capacity (FVC) —

5. Total lung capacity (TLC) —

D. Describe the method(s) by which each of these capacities are measured and give examples of diseases or conditions that may lead to a decrease or increase in the capacity.

1. Functional residual capacity —

2. Inspiratory capacity —

3. Vital capacity —

4. Forced vital capacity —

5. Total lung capacity —

E. Which capacity is used to measure flow studies such as FEV_1, $FEF_{25\%-75\%}$, and $FEF_{200-1200}$?

F. What is the normal RV/TLC ratio and give an example of a condition in which it is increased.

II. LUNG STUDIES

A. List four conditions in which minute volume would be increased.

1.

2.

3.

4.

B. What is the normal range for minute volume?

C. What ratio is the best indicator for distinguishing between an obstructive disorder and a restrictive one?

D. List the normal values for FEV/FVC ratio percentage in the following time periods:

_____ % of the FVC is exhaled in 0.5 second.

_____ % of the FVC is exhaled in 1 second.

_____ % of the FVC is exhaled in 2 seconds.

_____ % of the FVC is exhaled in 3 seconds.

E. Define forced expiratory volume.

F. Define $FEF_{200-1200}$ and give the normal value.

G. An FEV_1/FVC ratio of less than _____ indicates an obstructive disease.

H. Define $FEF_{25\%-75\%}$.

I. Define peak flow and give the normal value.

J. Define maximum voluntary ventilation (MVV) and explain its significance.

III. OBSTRUCTIVE VERSUS RESTRICTIVE DISEASES

A. List five obstructive diseases.

1.

2.

3.

4.

5.

B. What is the characteristic pulmonary function finding that determines an obstructive process?

C. List six restrictive diseases or disorders.

1.

2.

3.

4.

5.

6.

D. What is the characteristic pulmonary function finding that determines a restrictive process?

E. Pulmonary function predicted values are determined by what five factors?

1.

2.

3.

4.

5.

IV. MISCELLANEOUS PULMONARY FUNCTION STUDIES

A. What does a before-and-after bronchodilator study determine?

B. After a bronchodilator is administered, the flow studies must show an increase of at least
_____ % to prove significant reversibility of airway obstruction.

V. INTERPRETATION CHART SUMMARY

A. Determine if the following pulmonary function tests would be normal, increased, or decreased in an obstructive disorder:

1. FVC   Normal _____   Increased _____   Decreased _____

2. V_T Normal _____   Increased _____   Decreased _____

3. FRC   Normal _____   Increased _____   Decreased _____

4. RV   Normal _____   Increased _____   Decreased _____

5. RV/TLC   Normal _____   Increased _____   Decreased _____

6. FEV_1 Normal _____   Increased _____   Decreased _____

7. FEV/FVC   Normal _____   Increased _____   Decreased _____

8. $FEF_{25\%-75\%}$ Normal _____   Increased _____   Decreased _____

9. MVV   Normal _____   Increased _____   Decreased _____

B. Determine if the following pulmonary function tests would be normal, increased, or decreased in a restrictive disorder:

1. FVC   Normal _____   Increased _____   Decreased _____

2. V_T Normal _____   Increased _____   Decreased _____

3. FRC   Normal _____   Increased _____   Decreased _____

4. RV   Normal _____   Increased _____   Decreased _____

5. RV/TLC   Normal _____   Increased _____   Decreased _____

6. FEV_1 Normal _____   Increased _____   Decreased _____

7. FEV/FVC   Normal _____   Increased _____   Decreased _____

8. $FEF_{25\%-75\%}$ Normal _____   Increased _____   Decreased _____

9. MVV   Normal _____   Increased _____   Decreased _____

VI. FLOW-SENSING DEVICE

A. Describe the Wright respirometer and the purpose for which it is used.

CHAPTER 25

Entry-Level Respiratory Care Review Posttest

TIME LIMIT: 3 HOURS

Circle the best response.

The correct answers are found immediately following the last page of the exam. Please do not refer to the answers until you have completed the exam in the allotted time. Take this exam just as you would take the NBRC Entry Level Examination. You may miss up to 35 questions and still receive a passing score.

1. Inadequate alveolar ventilation caused by an airway obstruction is an example of which type of hypoxia?

A. anemic hypoxia
B. histotoxic hypoxia
C. circulatory hypoxia
D. hypoxemic hypoxia

2. Retrolental fibroplasia (RLF) occurs primarily in

A. premature infants.
B. chronic lung patients.
C. elderly patients.
D. asthmatics.

3. A patient is brought to the emergency room suffering from smoke inhalation after being pulled from a burning house. What would you recommend to best determine the severity of the patient's smoke inhalation?

A. pulse oximeter
B. arterial blood gases
C. CO-oximeter
D. transcutaneous Pa_{O_2} monitoring

4. The physician has ordered an active 3-year-old to be placed on 40% oxygen. Which device would you recommend as being the most tolerable for this patient?

A. Venturi mask
B. oxygen tent
C. aerosol mask
D. simple oxygen mask

5. The ability of the patient to follow instructions would be indicated by which of the following?

A. orientation to person
B. performance of tasks when asked
C. ability to feed himself
D. awareness of time

6. The respiratory care practitioner enters a patient's room to give an IPPB treatment and finds the patient unresponsive and not breathing. After delivering two breaths, what should the practitioner do next?

A. Continue rescue breathing.
B. Give the IPPB treatment as ordered.
C. Begin chest compressions.
D. Check for a pulse.

7. To most effectively increase a patient's alveolar ventilation while on a ventilator in the control mode, you would recommend increasing which one of the following?

A. inspiratory flowrate
B. ventilator rate
C. tidal volume
D. sigh rate

8. If the respiratory care practitioner fails to preoxygenate a patient on a ventilator prior to endotracheal suctioning, the result may be

 I. hypercapnia.
 II. hypoxemia.
 III. hypertension.
 IV. bradycardia.
A. I only
B. I and II only
C. II and III only
D. II and IV only

9. The most reliable method of determining if a ventilator patient's lungs are getting stiffer and harder to ventilate is by measuring the

A. static lung compliance.
B. dynamic lung compliance.
C. spontaneous tidal volume.
D. Pa_{O_2}.

10. A respiratory care practitioner is called to the recovery room to transport a patient to the ICU. After attaching the regulator to the E cylinder, gas is heard leaking from the cylinder. The practitioner should do which of the following?

 I. Tighten all connections.
 II. Check the cylinder outlet for dust or debris.
 III. Lubricate the regulator connection.
 IV. Replace the washer between the cylinder and regulator connections.
A. I and II only
B. II and IV only
C. III and IV only
D. I, II, and IV only

11. If not cleaned properly, which of the following devices is most likely to contaminate a patient's airways with bacteria?

A. bubble humidifier
B. cascade humidifier
C. hydrosphere
D. heated jet nebulizer

12. A baffle is used on a nebulizer to

A. break the aerosol into smaller particles.
B. entrain room air.
C. alter oxygen concentration.
D. heat the gas above room temperature.

13. Which of the following ABG results would be indicative of a renal compensated respiratory acidosis?

A. pH — 7.26, Pco_2 — 60, Po_2 — 68, HCO_3 — 24, B.E. 0
B. pH — 7.42, Pco_2 — 39, Po_2 — 87, HCO_3 — 22, B.E. –2
C. pH — 7.25, Pco_2 — 61, Po_2 — 75, HCO_3 — 26, B.E. +3
D. pH — 7.37, Pco_2 — 58, Po_2 — 60, HCO_3 — 31, B.E. +7

14. The number of stages a pressure reducing valve has can be determined by

A. identifying its safety system.
B. determining if it is adjustable or preset.
C. counting the number of pop-off valves.
D. reading the pressure gauge.

15. The advantage(s) of low-pressure, high-volume endotracheal tube cuffs is (are)

 I. easier insertion into the airway.
 II. less occlusion to tracheal blood flow.
 III. improved distribution of alveolar air.
A. I only
B. II only
C. I and II only
D. II and III only

16. Tracheal secretions tend to dry in an intubated patient when inspired air has which of the following characteristics?

 I. an absolute humidity of 24 mg per liter of gas
 II. a water vapor pressure of 47 mm Hg
 III. 50 mg of particulate water per liter of gas
 IV. a relative humidity of 100% at 25°C
A. II only
B. I and III only
C. I and IV only
D. II and III only

17. It is important to monitor airway pressure in a mechanically ventilated patient because it best reflects

A. lung compliance.
B. Pa_{O_2}.
C. Pa_{CO_2}.
D. intracranial pressure.

18. When a patient is being ventilated in the control mode how may the Pa_{CO_2} be raised?

A. Increase the tidal volume.
B. Increase the F_{IO_2}.
C. Increase the mechanical dead space.
D. Decrease the F_{IO_2}.

19. A patient is being ventilated on a volume ventilator and the low-pressure alarm suddenly sounds. The corrective action would be to

A. suction the patient.
B. begin manual resuscitation.
C. increase the flow.
D. check to determine whether the patient is disconnected from the ventilator.

20. A patient has just been intubated and you want to determine if the endotracheal tube is in the proper position. How may this be achieved?

   I. percussion
   II. chest x-ray
   III. negative inspiratory force
   IV. auscultation
A. II only
B. I and II only
C. II and IV only
D. III and IV only

21. If vocal cord trauma is suspected following extubation, the patient would exhibit which of the following symptoms?

A. wheezing
B. rhonchi
C. stridor
D. rales

22. To prevent the obstruction of venous blood flow to the tracheal wall, E-T tube cuff pressure should not exceed

A. 5 mm Hg.
B. 10 mm Hg.
C. 20 mm Hg.
D. 25 mm Hg.

23. A postoperative, 46-year-old, 80-kg (176-lb) patient is breathing spontaneously at a rate of 30/min on an F_{IO_2} of 0.50. The following arterial blood gas results are obtained.

   pH — 7.29
   Pa_{CO_2} — 62 torr
   Pa_{O_2} — 64 torr
   HCO_3 — 29 mEq/L

Mechanical ventilation is instituted with a tidal volume of 800 ml and an F_{IO_2} of 0.5. The SIMV rate should be

A. 4/min.
B. 6/min.
C. 12/min.
D. 16/min.

24. The respiratory care practitioner is asked to deliver medication to a cystic fibrosis patient via a hand-held nebulizer. Which of the following should be recommended?

A. isoproterenol (Isuprel)
B. hypertonic saline
C. propylene glycol
D. acetylcysteine (Mucomyst)

25. The therapeutic use of oxygen may aid in accomplishing which of the following?

   I. decrease the work of breathing
   II. decrease myocardial work
   III. prevent ARDS
   IV. increase the patient's respiratory rate
A. I only
B. I and II only
C. II and III only
D. I, II, and IV only

26. Inspiratory stridor is the major clinical sign of

A. tracheal malacia.
B. tracheal stenosis.
C. glottic edema.
D. laryngotracheal web.

27. When extubating a patient, it is important to remove the tube

A. at maximal inspiration.
B. at end exhalation.
C. between breaths.
D. at the beginning of inspiration.

28. Ventilator-induced hyperventilation would be apparent in blood gases by

A. increased pH, decreased Pa_{CO_2}.
B. increased pH, increased Pa_{CO_2}.
C. decreased pH, increased Pa_{CO_2}.
D. decreased pH, decreased Pa_{CO_2}.

29. As inspired air reaches the carina, it should be 100% saturated at body temperature, which represents how many milligrams of water per liter of air?

A. 32
B. 44
C. 47
D. 54

30. Choose the correct statements concerning the ventilation of a patient with a closed head injury.

    I. The patient should be hypoventilated in order to maintain elevated ICP levels.
    II. Shorter-than-normal inspiratory times should be maintained on the ventilator.
    III. Pa_{CO_2} levels should be maintained at 25 to 30 torr.
    IV. Machine tidal volume should be set for 15 ml/kg of ideal body weight.

A. I and II only
B. II and III only
C. I, III, and IV only
D. II, III and IV only

31. The following data pertain to an adult being mechanically ventilated.

    Peak airway pressure — 50 cm H_2O
    Plateau pressure — 40 cm H_2O
    Tidal volume — 800 ml (0.8 L)
    PEEP — 10 cm H_2O
    On the basis of this information, this patient's static lung compliance is approximately which of the following?

A. 16 ml/cm H_2O
B. 20 ml/cm H_2O
C. 27 ml/cm H_2O
D. 37 ml/cm H_2O

32. A patient recovering postoperatively is being ventilated in the IMV mode. The patient has normal blood gases on 35% oxygen but is still drowsy. The respiratory care practitioner should recommend decreasing the

A. IMV rate.
B. inspiratory time.
C. tidal volume.
D. inspiratory flow.

33. You need to transport a patient on a nasal cannula running at 6 L/min. In order to ensure that the cylinder will last at least 1 hour, what is the minimum amount of pressure an E cylinder must contain?

A. 1000 psig
B. 1200 psig
C. 1400 psig
D. 1600 psig

34. Which statement(s) relating to uncompensated Thorpe tube flowmeters is (are) true?

    I. The Thorpe tube is pressurized to 50 psig when plugged into the gas outlet.
    II. The needle valve is located before the Thorpe tube.
    III. The float will jump up and come back down while the flowmeter is plugged into a wall outlet with the needle valve closed.
    IV. Back pressure into the Thorpe tube does not affect the flow reading.

A. I only
B. II only
C. II and III only
D. III and IV only

35. Which of these drugs is used to temporarily paralyze a patient to facilitate intubation?

A. atropine sulfate
B. succinylcholine (Anectine)
C. curare
D. pancuronium bromide

36. To begin the weaning process from the ventilator, a patient should be able to obtain a negative inspiratory force of at least

A. 10 cm H_2O.
B. 20 cm H_2O.
C. 30 cm H_2O.
D. 40 cm H_2O.

37. While making oxygen rounds, you discover that the 6-inch reservoir tubing on a T-piece (Briggs adaptor) setup has fallen off. What may result from this?

    I. Delivered F_{IO_2} would decrease.
    II. Delivered F_{IO_2} would increase.
    III. The patient would entrain room air during inspiration.

A. I only
B. II only
C. I and II only
D. I and III only

38. A patient has been paralyzed with pancuronium bromide (Pavulon) and is being mechanically ventilated. Which of the following ventilator monitoring alarms would be most important?

A. low pressure
B. high pressure
C. inspired gas temperature
D. I:E ratio

39. Use of the inspiratory plateau setting on a ventilator results in

   I. decreasing mean intrathoracic pressure.
   II. increasing diffusion of gases.
   III. decreasing atelectasis.
A. I only
B. II only
C. I and II only
D. II and III only

40. A patient with chronic obstructive pulmonary disease is in the emergency room and is complaining of shortness of breath. Arterial blood gas results on room air are:

pH — 7.31
Pa$_{CO_2}$ — 62 torr
Pa$_{O_2}$ — 44 torr
The most appropriate recommendation for oxygen therapy is which of the following?
A. simple mask at 10 L/min.
B. nonrebreathing mask at 12 L/min.
C. Venturi mask at 28%
D. nasal cannula at 6 L/min.

41. To minimize damage to the lining of the tracheal mucosa during endotracheal suctioning,

A. normal saline should be instilled.
B. the catheter should not be left in the trachea more than 5 seconds.
C. intermittent suction should be applied.
D. the patient should be hyperoxygenated.

42. Which of these devices would be most indicated in the treatment of a patient with large amounts of thick secretions?

A. bubble humidifier
B. impeller nebulizer
C. pass-over humidifier
D. ultrasonic nebulizer

43. Which of these devices is not a low-flow device?

A. nasal cannula
B. Venturi mask
C. partial rebreathing mask
D. simple oxygen mask

44. You are instructing a patient about the proper procedure for using a metered-dose inhaler (MDI). You would instruct the patient to activate the medication in the inhaler

A. just prior to inspiration.
B. just after inspiration has begun.
C. at the end of expiration.
D. after inhaling as deeply as possible.

45. On chest x-ray the carina is located at what level?

A. second rib
B. third rib
C. fourth rib
D. fifth rib

46. While suctioning through a patient's E-T tube, you begin to have difficulty removing the thick secretions. Which of the following is the appropriate measure to take?

A. Increase the suctioning pressure to −180 torr.
B. Use a larger suction catheter.
C. Apply continuous suction while withdrawing the catheter.
D. Instill saline prior to suctioning.

47. CPAP is appropriate treatment on patients with which of the following?

A. apnea
B. spontaneous respiration with intrapulmonary shunting
C. patients being mechanically ventilated
D. spontaneous respiration without hypoxemia

48. Which of these is not a late complication of a tracheostomy?

A. infection
B. air embolism
C. dysfunction of the swallowing process
D. airway obstruction

49. A flowmeter has a completely closed needle valve, and the float jumps when the flowmeter is plugged into a gas source. Which of the following can be concluded?

~~I. This is an uncompensated flowmeter.~~
II. It is a Thorpe tube flowmeter.
~~III. The needle valve is malfunctioning.~~
IV. It is back pressure compensated.

A. I and II only
B. II and III only
C. II and IV only
D. III and IV only

50. Smokers will commonly have carboxyhemoglobin (HbCO) levels as high as

A. 10%.
B. 20%.
C. 30%.
D. 40%.

51. The purulence of secretions is caused by
yellow

A. the type of invading organism.
B. the elevation of body temperature.
C. the accumulation of red blood cells at the site of infection.
D. the accumulation of white blood cells at the site of infection.

52. A respiratory care practitioner asking the patient to take a maximal deep breath and rapidly exhale to maximum exhalation would be measuring the patient's

A. FVC.
B. NIF.
C. RV.
D. MVV.

53. A 75-kg (165-lb) patient is being mechanically ventilated in the IMV mode and has the following arterial blood gas results:

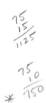

pH — 7.31
Pa$_{CO_2}$ — 59 torr
Pa$_{O_2}$ — 85 torr
HCO$_3$ — 29 mEq/L

The ventilator settings are as follows:

F$_{IO_2}$ — 0.35
IMV rate — 4/min.
Spontaneous rate — 24/min
Tidal volume — 600 ml

The respiratory care practitioner should recommend increasing which two of the following?

~~I. peak flowrate~~
II. IMV rate to 8/min
III. tidal volume to 750 ml
~~IV. F$_{IO_2}$ to 0.50~~

A. I and II
B. II and III
C. I and III
D. II and IV

54. The term "purulence" in reference to sputum means it is

A. yellow.
B. thick.
C. blood-streaked.
D. brown.

55. An oral endotracheal tube is inserted into an adult patient. An unusually large amount of air is needed to inflate the cuff. This problem could be caused by which of the following?

A. The E-T tube is too short.
B. The E-T tube is too long.
C. The E-T tube's inside diameter is too large.
D. The E-T tube's outside diameter is too small.

56. What is the most negative pressure that should supply the suction catheter when suctioning an adult?

A. –60 mm Hg
B. –80 mm Hg
C. –120 mm Hg
D. –160 mm Hg

57. Anatomic dead space is equal to   *150*

A. 1 ml/kg of body weight.
B. 5 ml/kg of body weight.
C. 1 ml/lb of body weight.
D. 3 ml/lb of body weight.

58. Subcutaneous emphysema is a condition resulting from

A. barotrauma.
B. emphysema.
C. decreased venous return.
D. decreased pulmonary blood flow.

59. A patient's Pa_{O_2} increased after the patient was placed on a ventilator at 21% oxygen. What accounts for the improved oxygenation status?

    I. increased distribution of ventilation
    II. increased dead space:tidal volume ratio
    III. decreased venous return to the heart
    IV. increased P(A–a) gradient

A. I only
B. I and II only
C. II and III only
D. II, III, and IV only

60. You enter a patient's room to administer a treatment and the patient is unresponsive. After opening the airway, what is the next appropriate measure to take?

A. Give two breaths.
B. Check for a pulse.
C. Deliver six abdominal thrusts.
D. Determine if the patient is breathing.

61. Which of the following are absolute contra-indications for IPPB therapy?

    I. tuberculosis
    II. untreated pneumothorax
    III. subcutaneous emphysema
    IV. pulmonary hemorrhage

A. I and II only
B. II and IV only
C. III and IV only
D. I, II, and III only

62. During the administration of IPPB with the Bird Mark 7, the respiratory care practitioner notices the machine repeatedly cycles on shortly after the patient has begun expiration. In order to correct this problem the practitioner should check which of the following controls?

A. flow control
B. peak pressure control
C. sensitivity control
D. air mix control

63. A nasopharyngeal airway has which of the following advantages?

    I. It will ensure lower airway patency during mechanical ventilation.
    II. It provides an adequate route for laryngo-tracheal suctioning.
    III. It is well tolerated by the semicomatose patient.

A. I only
B. II only
C. I and II only
D. II and III only

64. If you choose an E cylinder to transport a patient within the hospital and it contains 650 psig of oxygen, how long will the cylinder last if you run the flow at 10 L/min?

A. 18 minutes
B. 35 minutes
C. 56 minutes
D. 1 hour, 45 minutes

65. Which of these airway changes will affect the delivered tidal volume on a pressure-limited ventilator?

    I. decreased lung compliance
    II. increased lung compliance
    III. increased airway resistance

A. I only
B. I and II only
C. I and III only
D. I, II, and III

66. The respiratory care practitioner should recommend which of the following first, for a patient with a tension pneumothorax.

A. Obtain a stat chest x-ray.
B. Obtain a stat arterial blood gas.
C. Administer IPPB.
D. Release air from the pleural space.

67. A COPD patient breathing spontaneously on an $F_{I_{O_2}}$ of 0.6 becomes drowsy and unresponsive. The patient's reaction is most likely the result of

A. insufficient oxygenation.
B. decreased venous return.
C. increased Pa_{CO_2}.
D. excessive ventilation.

68. While performing chest wall percussion on a ventilator patient, you notice an area of hyper-resonance. This is diagnostic for which of the following conditions?

A. pleural effusion
B. pneumothorax
C. pulmonary edema
D. consolidation

69. A patient's pulse drops from 92 to 54 per minute when a suction catheter is inserted into the oropharynx. The most likely cause is

A. hypoxia.
B. vagal stimulation.
C. hypocapnia.
D. coughing.

70. Inspired air is humidified primarily by

A. nasal structures.
B. alveoli.
C. the larynx.
D. cilia.

71. A nebulizer is used to

A. warm inspired gas.
B. decrease gas density.
C. increase the partial pressure of the gas.
D. facilitate secretion removal.

72. You have been asked to deliver a low percentage of oxygen to a patient that is breathing 30 times a minute with an irregular breathing pattern. Which device would be the best choice?

A. nasal cannula at 2 L/min
B. Venturi mask at 28%
C. simple oxygen mask at 5 L/min
D. nasal catheter at 1 L/min

73. Which of the following blood gas results would be considered normal on a severe COPD patient?

A. pH — 7.28, P_{CO_2} — 40 torr, P_{O_2} — 56 torr, HCO_3 — 30 mEq/L
B. pH — 7.56, P_{CO_2} — 28 torr, P_{O_2} — 60 torr, HCO_3 — 28 mEq/L
C. pH — 7.36, P_{CO_2} — 40 torr, P_{O_2} — 85 torr, HCO_3 — 24 mEq/L
D. pH — 7.38, P_{CO_2} — 60 torr, P_{O_2} — 57 torr, HCO_3 — 33 mEq/L

74. Normal I:E ratio for an adult is

A. 1:1.
B. 2:1.
C. 1:2.
D. 1:5.

75. Which of the following is not a hazard of IPPB?

A. decreased cardiac output
B. increased venous blood return
C. excessive ventilation
D. gastric insufflation

76. The oropharyngeal airway

I. can be inserted orally or nasally.
II. can cause activation of the gag reflex.
III. is more suitable for conscious patients.

A. I only
B. II only
C. I and II only
D. II and III only

77. What is the most appropriate ventilator tidal volume setting for a 65-kg (143-lb) patient.

A. 350 ml
B. 500 ml
C. 650 ml
D. 1000 ml

78. Which of the following parameters, when changed, will alter the inspiratory time on a volume-limited ventilator?

I. rate control
II. flowrate control
III. tidal volume control
IV. expiratory resistance control

A. I and II only
B. II and III only
C. II and IV only
D. I, II, and III only

79. Which of the following situations would result in activation of the high-pressure alarm on a volume-limited ventilator?

I. leak in the circuit
II. patient disconnected from the ventilator
III. patient coughing
IV. water in the tubing

A. I and III only
B. II and IV only
C. III and IV only
D. I, III, and IV only

80. Which statement concerning the inspiratory hold control on a volume-limited ventilator is true?

A. It may be utilized to improve oxygenation.
B. It may be utilized to decrease Pa_{CO_2} levels.
C. It lengthens expiratory time.
D. It is used to calculate tubing compliance.

81. While making oxygen rounds, you notice the mist coming out of the exhalation ports of a patient's aerosol mask completely disappears as the patient inspires. What should be recommended at this time?

A. Add a heater to the nebulizer.
B. Make sure the mask is a tight fit.
C. Increase the flow from the nebulizer.
D. Replace the aerosol mask with a face tent.

82. A patient with diabetes enters the emergency room breathing very deeply and rapidly. This type of breathing pattern is called

A. Kussmaul's respiration.
B. Biot's respiration.
C. Cheyne-Stokes respiration.
D. hypopnea.

83. On chest x-ray film you notice the patient's E-T tube is resting at the level of the fifth rib. The tube most likely entered the

A. left mainstem bronchus.
B. right mainstem bronchus.
C. esophagus.
D. right upper lobe bronchiole.

84. The polarographic electrode is used in which type of oxygen analyzer?

A. chemical analyzer
B. physical analyzer
C. electric analyzer
D. electrochemical analyzer

85. The polarographic oxygen analyzer being used to analyze a patient's aerosol mask is reading inaccurately. Which of the following would not result in this inaccurate reading?

A. no electrolyte gel
B. torn membrane
C. water on the membrane
D. dead fuel cell

86. Which of the following are capable of sterilizing equipment?

   I. autoclave
   II. ethylene oxide
   III. glutaraldehyde
   IV. alcohols
A. I and II only
B. II and III only
C. I and IV only
D. I, II, and III only

87. Assuming a patient has an ideal breathing pattern, what is the maximum percentage of oxygen delivered with a nasal cannula at 6 L/min?

A. 28%
B. 36%
C. 44%
D. 52%

88. Most bubble humidifiers produce a body humidity of about

A. 10% to 20%.
B. 30% to 40%.
C. 50% to 60%.
D. 70% to 80%.

89. After turning the oxygen flowmeter completely off, you notice the water in the humidifier is still slightly bubbling. What is the most likely reason for this?

A. The humidifier lid is not tight.
B. There is a crack in the humidifier jar.
C. The wall outlet is loose.
D. There is a faulty valve seat in the flowmeter.

90. DISS connections are used with gas administration equipment that operates at

A. 200 psig or less.
B. 500 psig or less.
C. 1000 psig.
D. 2200 psig.

91. A patient has been experiencing a moderate asthmatic attack for 30 minutes. Which of the following arterial blood gas results would you expect to observe if the patient was on room air?

A. pH — 7.42, Pa_{CO_2} — 44 torr, Pa_{O_2} — 81 torr
B. pH — 7.08, Pa_{CO_2} — 74 torr, Pa_{O_2} — 50 torr
C. pH — 7.51, Pa_{CO_2} — 27 torr, Pa_{O_2} — 60 torr
D. pH — 7.55, Pa_{CO_2} — 22 torr, Pa_{O_2} — 93 torr

92. Therapy is ordered for a patient producing large amounts of thick, purulent secretions. What device should the respiratory care practitioner recommend?

A. ultrasonic nebulizer
B. hand-held nebulizer
C. cascade humidifier
D. impeller nebulizer

93. If a patient's Pa_{CO_2} decreases to 27 torr, all of the following could have increased except

A. physiologic dead space.
B. alveolar ventilation.
C. respiratory rate.
D. minute ventilation.

94. Which of the following devices should be recommended for a patient brought into the emergency room suffering from smoke inhalation?

A. Venturi mask
B. nasal cannula
C. simple oxygen mask
D. nonrebreathing mask

95. Hazards associated with aerosol therapy include all of the following except

A. fluid overload in infants.
B. bronchospasm.
C. swelling of dried, retained secretions.
D. bradycardia.

96. If a small hole is present in the exhalation valve diaphragm of an IPPB circuit, the machine will

A. automatically cycle into exhalation.
B. cycle into exhalation prematurely on each breath.
C. deliver an increased inspiratory pressure to the patient.
D. not cycle into expiration.

97. Which of the following organisms is most frequently cultured from heated nebulizers and humidifiers?

A. *Staphylococcus aureus*
B. *Pseudomonas aeruginosa*
C. *Mycobacterium tuberculosis*
D. *Serratia marcescens*

98. Which of these are causes of glottic edema?

  I. traumatic intubation
  II. overinflated E-T tube cuff
  III. oversized E-T tube
  IV. allergic response to material in the E-T tube
A. I and II only
B. II and III only
C. I and III only
D. I, III, and IV only

99. Chest physiotherapy is indicated in all of the following except

A. pulmonary edema.
B. bronchiectasis.
C. cystic fibrosis.
D. aspiration pneumonia.

100. The respiratory care practitioner is administering IPPB therapy to a postoperative patient using a mouthpiece. During the treatment, the patient is unable to cycle the machine off. What could be done to correct this problem?

  I. Check for a leak in the system.
  II. Check the exhalation valve function.
  III. Decrease the cycling pressure to 10 cm H_2O.
  IV. Adjust the sensitivity.
A. I only
B. III only
C. I and II only
D. II and IV only

101. Which of the following are physiologic effects of IPPB therapy?

  I. decreased mean airway pressure
  II. increased tidal volume
  III. improved distribution of ventilation
  IV. mechanical bronchodilation
A. I and II only
B. II and III only
C. II, III, and IV only
D. I, II, and IV only

102. A postoperative patient is to be treated for the prevention of atelectasis. The patient is still heavily sedated. Which type of therapy should be recommended?

A. blow bottles
B. incentive spirometry
C. hand-held nebulizer
D. IPPB

103. Which of the following can be determined from a forced expiratory spirogram?

  I. FEV_1
  II. $FEF_{200-1200}$ *Large airways*
  III. functional residual capacity *Not FRC*
A. I only
B. II only
C. I and II only
D. II and III only

104. A COPD patient is admitted with fever, cough, and mild confusion. Oxygen is administered via a nasal cannula at 3 L/min. One-half hour later, the patient is less alert. Arterial blood gas analysis is as follows:

Room Air on Admission	*Nasal Cannula (3 L/min)*
pH — 7.30	pH — 7.19
Pa_{CO_2} — 65 torr	Pa_{CO_2} — 76 torr
HCO_3 — 34 mEq/L	HCO_3 — 33 mEq/L
Pa_{O_2} — 36 torr	Pa_{O_2} — 46 torr

The most appropriate change in the patient's treatment would be to

A. use a 28% Venturi mask.
B. use a simple mask at 12 L/min.
C. decrease the oxygen flow.
D. institute mechanical ventilation with an F_{IO_2} of 0.4.

105. A nebulizer is set on the 40% dilution mode and connected to an oxygen flowmeter running at 12 L/min. What is the total flow output of this nebulizer?

A. 24 L/min
B. 36 L/min
C. 48 L/min
D. 54 L/min

106. A patient on mechanical ventilation has the following arterial blood gas values:

pH — 7.56
Pa_{CO_2} — 22 torr
HCO_3 — 24 mEq/L
Pa_{O_2} — 102 torr

All of the following ventilator changes would help correct this *except*

A. decreasing respiratory rate.
B. increasing tidal volume.
C. placement on IMV.
D. adding mechanical dead space.

107. Assuming the patient has an ideal breathing pattern, what is the approximate oxygen percentage delivered with a nasal cannula at 2 L/min?

A. 24%
B. 28%
C. 32%
D. 36%

108. For a patient with a tidal volume of 450 ml and a respiratory rate that fluctuates between 15 and 25 breaths per minute, which of the following is the best device for the administration of a controlled oxygen percentage?

A. partial rebreathing mask
B. simple oxygen mask
C. Venturi mask
D. nasal cannula

109. Which of these arterial blood gases would be most beneficial to a patient on a ventilator with a closed head injury?

A. pH — 7.59, P_{CO_2} — 18 torr, P_{O_2} — 90 torr
B. pH — 7.25, P_{CO_2} — 55 torr, P_{O_2} — 50 torr
C. pH — 7.44, P_{CO_2} — 40 torr, P_{O_2} — 80 torr
D. pH — 7.52, P_{CO_2} — 28 torr, P_{O_2} — 94 torr

110. If a patient on a ventilator is set up in such a way for the inverse I:E ratio alarm to be activated, what ventilator change could be made to correct this breathing pattern?

A. Decrease flowrate.
B. Increase flowrate.
C. Increase tidal volume.
D. Increase respiratory rate.

111. While preparing to analyze a patient's aerosol mask, you notice water in the tubing. What effect would this have on the operation of this device?

A. decrease the F_{IO_2}
B. increase the F_{IO_2}
C. increase air entrainment into the nebulizer
D. increase gas flow to the patient

112. Which of the following are considered reasons for providing aerosol to the patient's airway?

I. mobilization of retained secretions
II. overhydration
III. induce sputum
IV. deliver bronchodilator
V. soothe irritated airways following extubation

A. I, II, and III only
B. II, IV, and V only
C. I, III, IV, and V only
D. II, III, IV, and V only

113. To minimize an increased airway resistance produced by high-density aerosol inhalation, the respiratory care practitioner should

A. use a bronchodilator in conjunction with the aerosol.
B. instruct the patient to breathe through the nose.
C. always use a heated aerosol.
D. perform chest physiotherapy following the aerosol treatment.

114. A patient's heated nebulizer is delivering 41 mg of water/liter of gas. The percentage of body humidity delivered by this device is

A. 32%.
B. 41%.
C. 64%.
D. 93%.

p 38

$$\frac{41}{44} \cdot 100 = 93\%$$

115. A volume of air at 22°C can hold 19 mg of water/liter of gas. What is the relative humidity of the gas if it is holding 14 mg of water/liter of gas?

A. 14%
B. 21%
C. 43%
D. 74%

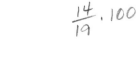

$$\frac{14}{19} \cdot 100$$

116. Which of the following aerosol generators (nebulizers) depends on the effects of lateral negative pressure to pull fluid over a sphere so it may be exposed to a high-velocity jet?

A. pneumatic jet
B. spinning disk
C. ultrasonic
D. Babington

117. A patient with a broken nose and cheekbone is to be placed on 40% oxygen. The patient's secretions are thick. Based on this information, which oxygen delivery device would be indicated?

A. nasal cannula at 5 L/min
B. face tent
C. simple oxygen mask at 8 L/min
D. aerosol mask

118. An order is written by the physician to place a patient on a 40% aerosol mask. You want to achieve a total flow of at least 40 L/min. What would be the minimum flow setting on the flowmeter to achieve this total flow?

A. 6 L/min
B. 8 L/min
C. 10 L/min
D. 12 L/min

119. Which piece of equipment is most commonly used for the setup of a tracheostomy collar?

A. bubble humidifier
B. impeller nebulizer
C. ultrasonic nebulizer
D. jet nebulizer

120. Choose the device that is not connected to a humidifier.

A. simple oxygen mask
B. T-piece (Briggs adaptor)
C. partial rebreathing mask
D. nonrebreathing mask

121. Which of the following respiratory medications is not considered a bronchodilator?

A. Alupent
B. Bronkosol
C. Terbutaline
D. Mucomyst

122. A patient is breathing 16 times per minute and has a tidal volume of 450 ml. What is this patient's minute ventilation?

A. 4.2 L
B. 6.1 L
C. 7.2 L
D. 8.6 L

123. A patient is breathing spontaneously on a 60% aerosol mask with the following arterial blood gas results:

pH — 7.36
P_{CO_2} — 43 torr
HCO_3 — 24 mEq/L
P_{O_2} — 48 torr

Based on this information, the respiratory care practitioner should recommend which of the following?

A. Place on CPAP.
B. Increase oxygen percentage to 80%.
C. Place on nonrebreathing mask.
D. Intubate and place on tidal volume of 800 ml.

124. A patient is being mechanically ventilated on the following settings:

Tidal volume — 750 ml
Respiratory rate — 12/min
Mode — assist-control
PEEP — 10 cm H_2O
F_{IO_2} — 0.60

Arterial blood gas results on these settings are:

pH — 7.41
P_{CO_2} — 38 torr
P_{O_2} — 174 torr

Based on the above information, what would be the appropriate ventilator change?

A. Decrease PEEP.
B. Decrease F_{IO_2}.
C. Increase mechanical dead space.
D. Decrease tidal volume.

125. The reduction in urinary output caused by mechanical ventilation is due to

I. decreased renal blood flow.
II. decreased production of antidiuretic hormone (ADH).
III. increased pulmonary blood flow.
IV. increased renal blood flow.
V. increased production of antidiuretic hormone (ADH).

A. I and V only
B. II and III only
C. I, III, and V only
D. I, II, and IV only

126. Which values would most likely indicate that a patient may be weaned from mechanical ventilation?

    I. VD/VT ratio of .45
    II. NIF of 28 cm H_2O
    III. P(A–a) gradient of 500 mm Hg on 100% oxygen
    IV. Vital capacity of 16 ml/kg

A. I and II only
B. II and III only
C. I, II, and IV only
D. II, III, and IV only

127. Where should a respirometer be placed to most accurately determine the volume being delivered by a ventilator?

A. at the ventilator outlet ✓
B. at the exhalation valve
C. between the patient's E-T tube and the ventilator wye
D. at the humidifier outlet

128. A patient is being mechanically ventilated on a volume-cycled ventilator in the control mode. The low pressure alarm is sounding. This may be the result of which one of the following?

A. Water in the tubing.
B. Patient disconnected from the ventilator.
C. Secretions in the patient's airway.
D. Kink in the ventilator tubing.

129. The peak inspiratory pressure has dropped from 34 cm H_2O to 10 cm H_2O on a volume-limited ventilator operating in the control mode. You notice the expired volume spirometer is filling during inspiration. Which of the following would be the most likely cause of this problem?

A. There is a leak in the endotracheal tube cuff.
B. There is a malfunction of the exhalation valve.
C. There is a malfunction of the pressure manometer.
D. The inspiratory flowrate is set too high.

130. You have just obtained blood from the patient's radial artery to determine arterial blood gas results. As you run the blood through the blood gas analyzer you notice you failed to remove an air bubble from the sample. The blood gas results will most likely reflect values with a

A. high pH and low PO_2.
B. low PCO_2 and low PO_2.
C. low PCO_2 and high PO_2. *air bubble*
D. high PCO_2 and high PO_2.

131. The respiratory care practitioner is monitoring a patient with Guillain-Barré syndrome for respiratory impairment. Which of the following parameters would provide the earliest determination?

A. Pa_{O_2}
B. Pa_{CO_2}
C. maximal inspiratory pressure
D. FVC

Questions 132–134 concern the following situation:

A 36-year-old, 65-kg (143-lb) unconscious man is admitted to the emergency room. His breathing rate is 8/min and very shallow. A drug overdose is suspected.

132. To maintain a patent airway, what type of device should be employed?

A. nasal catheter
B. bite block
C. oropharyngeal airway
D. tongue depressor

133. The patient becomes apneic and mechanical ventilatory support is required. How would the airway best be maintained?

A. fenestrated tracheostomy tube
B. CPAP mask
C. cuffed endotracheal tube
D. uncuffed endotracheal tube

134. The most appropriate ventilator settings would be which of the following?

A. tidal volume — 600 ml, rate — 10, control mode
B. tidal volume — 800 ml, rate — 6, control mode
C. CPAP — 4 cm H_2O
D. tidal volume — 700 ml, rate — 12, control mode

Questions 135–137 concern the following situation:

A 48-year-old, 75-kg (165-lb) woman is in the intensive care unit following coronary bypass surgery. The patient has been ordered to be placed on mechanical ventilation.

135. As you connect the patient to the ventilator, you notice the peak inspiratory pressure is registering 10 cm H_2O on the manometer and the exhaled volume spirometer is showing 300 ml less than the

volume setting. Which of the following could be causing this problem? _leak_

    I.   There is a leak around the cascade humidifier.

    II. The medication nebulizer is not connected tightly.

    ~~III. There is no water in the cascade humidifier.~~

A. I only

B. II only

C. I and II only

D. II and III only

136. During ventilator checks 6 hours later, you notice the peak inspiratory pressure has been gradually increasing. What could be the cause?

    I.   bronchospasm

    II. accumulation of secretions

    ~~III. increasing pulmonary compliance~~

    ~~IV. decreasing airway resistance~~

A. I and II only

B. II and IV only

C. III and IV only

D. I, II, III, and IV

137. The following day, the patient is placed on T-tube flow-by for weaning purposes. During this time, the patient's respiratory rate increases to 30/min and her blood pressure begins to drop. What is the appropriate measure to take at this time?

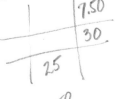

A. Place on IMV rate of 8.

B. Obtain stat chest x-ray.

C. Place on CPAP.

D. Place on control mode, rate of 10.

Questions 138–140 concern the following situation:

A 17-year-old boy is admitted to the emergency room with multiple rib fractures following a motor vehicle accident. An arterial blood gas measurement reveals the following results on room air:

pH — 7.50

P_{CO_2} — 30 torr

HCO_3 — 25 mEq/L

P_{O_2} — 58 torr

138. These data indicate which of the following?

    ~~I. decreased P(A–a) gradient~~

    II. hyperventilation

    ~~III. respiratory acidosis~~

A. I only

B. II only

C. I and II only

D. II and III only

139. The patient's condition has worsened and mechanical ventilation is initiated. What parameters should the practitioner determine at this time?

    I.   tidal volume required by patient

    ~~II. patient's FVC~~

    ~~III. patient's negative inspiratory force~~

    IV. minute ventilation required by patient

A. I and II only

B. I and IV only

C. I, II, and IV only

D. I, II, III, and IV

140. Six days later, the physician is considering weaning this patient from the ventilator. The following data are collected:

NIF — –30 cm H_2O

VC — 3.0 L

Arterial blood gases on 35% oxygen reveal:

pH — 7.38

P_{CO_2} — 41 torr

HCO_3 — 25 mEq/L

P_{O_2} — 86 torr

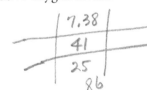

Based on the above information, the practitioner should recommend which of the following?

A. Institute IMV.

B. Continue mechanical ventilation on assist-control.

C. Increase the tidal volume.

D. Add mechanical dead space.

POSTTEST ANSWERS

Following each answer is the study guide chapter where information concerning the answer may be found.

1. D	Ch. 2	38. A	Ch. 9	75. B	Ch. 6	108. C	Ch. 2		
2. A	Ch. 2	39. D	Ch. 9	76. B	Ch. 5	109. D	Ch. 9		
3. C	Ch. 2	40. C	Ch. 10	77. C	Ch. 9	110. B	Ch. 9		
4. B	Ch. 2	41. C	Ch. 5	78. B	Ch. 9	111. B	Ch. 3		
5. B	Ch. 1	42. D	Ch. 3	79. C	Ch. 9	112. C	Ch. 3		
6. D	Ch. 7	43. B	Ch. 2	80. A	Ch. 9	113. A	Ch. 3		
7. C	Ch. 9	44. B	Ch. 3	81. C	Ch. 2	114. D	Ch. 3		
8. D	Ch. 5	45. C	Ch. 5	82. A	Ch. 1	115. D	Ch. 3		
9. A	Ch. 9	46. D	Ch. 5	83. B	Ch. 4	116. D	Ch. 3		
10. D	Ch. 2	47. B	Ch. 9	84. D	Ch. 2	117. B	Ch. 2		
11. D	Ch. 3	48. B	Ch. 5	85. D	Ch. 2	118. C	Ch. 2		
12. A	Ch. 3	49. C	Ch. 2	86. D	Ch. 4	119. D	Ch. 2		
13. D	Ch. 8	50. A	Ch. 2	87. C	Ch. 2	120. B	Ch. 2		
14. C	Ch. 2	51. D	Ch. 1	88. B	Ch. 3	121. D	Ch. 11		
15. B	Ch. 5	52. A	Ch. 12	89. D	Ch. 2	122. C	Ch. 9		
16. C	Ch. 3	53. B	Ch. 9	90. A	Ch. 2	123. A	Ch. 9		
17. A	Ch. 9	54. A	Ch. 1	91. C	Ch. 10	124. A	Ch. 9		
18. C	Ch. 9	55. D	Ch. 5	92. A	Ch. 3	125. A	Ch. 9		
19. D	Ch. 9	56. C	Ch. 5	93. A	Ch. 8	126. C	Ch. 9		
20. C	Ch. 5	57. C	Ch. 9	94. D	Ch. 2	127. A	Ch. 9		
21. C	Ch. 5	58. A	Ch. 9	95. D	Ch. 3	128. B	Ch. 9		
22. C	Ch. 5	59. A	Ch. 9	96. D	Ch. 6	129. B	Ch. 9		
23. C	Ch. 9	60. D	Ch. 7	97. B	Ch. 3	130. C	Ch. 8		
24. D	Ch. 11	61. B	Ch. 6	98. D	Ch. 5	131. C	Ch. 9		
25. B	Ch. 2	62. C	Ch. 6	99. A	Ch. 5	132. C	Ch. 5		
26. C	Ch. 5	63. D	Ch. 5	100. C	Ch. 6	133. C	Ch. 5		
27. A	Ch. 5	64. A	Ch. 2	101. C	Ch. 6	134. D	Ch. 9		
28. A	Ch. 8	65. D	Ch. 9	102. D	Ch. 6	135. C	Ch. 9		
29. B	Ch. 3	66. D	Ch. 10	103. C	Ch. 12	136. A	Ch. 9		
30. B	Ch. 9	67. C	Ch. 10	104. D	Ch. 10	137. A	Ch. 9		
31. C	Ch. 9	68. B	Ch. 1	105. C	Ch. 2	138. B	Ch. 8		
32. A	Ch. 9	69. B	Ch. 5	106. B	Ch. 8	139. B	Ch. 9		
33. C	Ch. 2	70. A	Ch. 3	107. B	Ch. 2	140. A	Ch. 9		
34. B	Ch. 2	71. D	Ch. 3						
35. B	Ch. 11	72. B	Ch. 2						
36. B	Ch. 9	73. D	Ch. 8						
37. D	Ch. 2	74. C	Ch. 9						

CHAPTER **26**

Taking the
Examination

This section is to provide you with helpful hints that should improve your test-taking skills and confidence level prior to taking the NBRC Entry-Level Certification Examination.

1. Memorize as few math formulas as possible.

The examination may require you to calculate answers to commonly used math formulas but add a little twist to the question. Calculating how long the contents of an E cylinder of oxygen will last before the cylinder runs empty is relatively simple because it is done so often. Commonly, the liter flow and pressure in the cylinder is given, and you only need to know the cylinder factor and the equation (see Section II, "Oxygen and Medical Gas Therapy").

But what if the exam asks the question in the following manner?

The respiratory care practitioner is transporting a patient on oxygen from ICU to radiology. The patient is on a 4 L/min nasal cannula. The practitioner wants to make sure the E cylinder chosen for transport has enough gas to last at least 1 hour. What is the minimum pressure the cylinder must contain?

A. 400 psig
B. 600 psig
C. 800 psig
D. 1000 psig

Don't let questions such as these make you panic. It is not necessary to know another math equation in order to work this problem. You may still use the common equation:

$$\text{minutes remaining in the cylinder} = \frac{\text{cylinder pressure} \times \text{cylinder factor}}{\text{liter flow}}$$

Simply insert each answer given (A to D), *starting with the "C" choice,* into the equation and pick the pressure that allows for at least 1 hour of running time. Start with the "C" choice so you will not have to try more than two choices.

For the question above, insert 800 psig ("C" choice) into the equation you already know.

$$\frac{800 \text{ psig} \times 0.28}{4 \text{ L/min}} = 56 \text{ minutes}$$

Because 56 minutes is less than 1 hour, you know the correct answer must be greater than 800 psig. The answer must be choice "D" (1000 psig).

$$\frac{1000 \text{ psig} \times 0.28}{4 \text{ L/min}} = 70 \text{ minutes}$$

Another common formula is used to calculate total flow delivered by a high-flow oxygen device or nebulizer. By adding the air:oxygen entrainment ratio parts together and multiplying by the flowrate, we can calculate total flow (see Section II, "Oxygen and Medical Gas Therapy").

But what if the question is asked as follows:

A patient on a 40% aerosol mask has an inspiratory flowrate of 42 L/min. What is the minimum oxygen flowmeter setting needed in order to meet this patient's inspiratory flow demands?

A. 8 L/min
B. 10 L/min
C. 12 L/min
D. 14 L/min

Again, start with the "C" choice (12 L/min) and multiply it by the total air:oxygen ratio parts for 40% (3:1) or 4.

$$4 \times 12 = 48 \text{ L/min}$$

This meets and even exceeds the patient's 42 L/min flow demand. But to make sure 12 L/min is the minimum flow required, check the "B" choice (10 L/min).

$$4 \times 10 = 40 \text{ L/min}$$

The flow setting for the "B" choice is too low (40 L/min), so the correct flow setting is 12 L/min or the "C" choice.

Remember, you are not allowed to use a calculator when taking the exam. Therefore, it is important not to waste time doing calculations. I think this test-taking strategy will both save time and limit the number of equations you need to remember for the exam.

Some people have stated with tongue in cheek that all the correct answers are on a multiple-choice test. This statement is, of course, true. The problem is identifying which choice is correct. Use this to your advantage in the problems we have just worked. You know that one of the choices is correct. Simply plug it into the equation with which you are most familiar and you should be able to avoid wasting time and answer the question correctly.

2. **How to simplify the multiple multiple-choice question.**

Of all the questions on the Entry-Level Examination, I think the most intimidating one is the multiple multiple-choice question, sometimes called the multiple true/false question.

An example of this type of question is as follows:

Which of the following oxygen delivery devices are considered high-flow devices?

   I. Venturi mask
  II. nasal cannula
 III. aerosol mask
 IV. simple oxygen mask

A. I and II only
B. I and III only
C. II and IV only
D. I, III, and IV only

This question may not be as difficult as it seems. If you are sure that one or two of the devices are high-flow or low-flow, you can greatly improve your chances of getting this question correct.

For instance, if you know that an aerosol mask is a high-flow device, then you know the correct answer must include "III" (aerosol mask). This rules out choice "A" and "C."

This reduces your choices to two instead of four. You have increased the possibility of answering this question correctly. You may say you are guessing on this question, but it is an educated guess because you have ruled out answers you know to be incorrect.

This process of elimination has reduced your choices to "B" and "D," a 50-50 chance of correctly answering this question. You now have a much higher probability of getting this question right without having to know everything about high- and low-flow oxygen delivery devices.

You will see quite a few multiple multiple-choice questions on the Entry-Level Examination. Do not be intimidated. Look for at least one choice you are sure of and, as you have seen, this can greatly increase your chances of getting these types of questions correct.

3. **Don't spend too much time on one question.**

One mistake many people make while taking the exam is spending too much time on a particular question. If this happens on several questions, you may find yourself running out of time and not able to spend time on questions you may know. If you are having difficulty making a choice, rule out the choices you know are wrong and make an educated guess. Go on to the next question and do not give the previous question another thought. You may make a mark in the test booklet as a reminder to return to the question after you have finished the test if you feel it is needed. Change your answer only if you know for certain the choice you made is wrong. Many times the first choice is the correct one.

4. Read the question and all of the answer choices carefully.

I cannot emphasize this enough. You will see questions on the exam that ask you to choose which one does not apply. For example, the question may state, "All of the following are true except...." This can be confusing. As you begin looking at the choices, you may forget you are looking for the *false* choice and choose a true choice, of which there are three. We are accustomed to choosing true statements for the correct answer. It is a good idea to read the question two or three times to make sure it is asking you to choose a false response.

Also, make sure that you read all four of the choices, even if you feel certain that a particular choice is correct. You may be wrong. Here is an example:

You enter a patient's room and find the patient unconscious and not breathing. What should the respiratory care practitioner do first?

A. Give the patient two breaths.
B. Check for a pulse.
C. Administer a precordial thump.
D. Open the patient's airway.

Some people would choose "A" and never look at the rest of the choices. Look at the "D" choice. This is the correct answer, and some would never have seen it. The "A" choice sounds good, but it is not the correct answer.

Remember, too, that some questions may have an "acceptable" answer (which is not the right answer) and a "correct" answer. Make sure you look at all the choices so you will have at least seen the "correct" answer.

5. Check your answer sheet periodically.

Make sure the number you are marking on your answer sheet corresponds to the question number in the test booklet. Getting off-number can be disastrous.

6. Prepare a planned study schedule.

Prepare for the exam by beginning regular study sessions several weeks before the exam. Study at least 1 hour each day for five days each week.

Begin with Chapter One in the study guide section by answering the pretest questions. Grade your answers by looking at the answer sheet on the last page of the chapter. Proceed to study each page in this chapter until it is finished. Turn to the workbook section and answer as many questions as you can without looking back to the study guide section. When you have finished answering all the questions you can, return to the unanswered questions, look them up in the study guide section, and record the answers in the workbook. Pay special attention to the questions you could not answer. Go back and check the answers you have recorded in the workbook section and make sure they are correct. Any incorrect answers should be corrected in the workbook.

Longer chapters will take more than 1 hour to complete, but try to complete one chapter per day. Do not rush through the material. Take your time and absorb as much as you can. If you begin to tire, stop. Continue the study session after a brief break or the next day.

Continue through the study guide and workbook sections chapter by chapter until you have completed each one. After you are finished, set aside one 3-hour period to take the posttest in the back of the workbook section. Take it as though it is the actual exam. After completion of the posttest, grade it using the answer sheet on the page immediately following the test. Note that after each answer on the answer sheet there is the chapter from the study guide where information concerning this answer can be found. Go back and look up the questions that you answered incorrectly, making note of your weakest areas. It is these areas you should study more extensively.

Those who receive this book only 2 or 3 weeks prior to the Entry-Level Certification Examination will have to alter the previously mentioned study schedule. You may need to do two chapters per day to finish the study guide/workbook.

I recommend not studying the night before the examination. This may cause stress as you realize you do not know all of the material. You will not learn it all by studying all night anyway. Remember, you don't have to have all the correct answers, only 75% of them. It is important to get a good night's sleep and feel refreshed the morning of the test.

It is my hope and prayer that by using this book as it is intended and using the test-taking skills mentioned in this chapter, you will successfully complete the NBRC Entry-Level Certification Examination.

INDEX

Note: Page numbers in *italics* refer to illustrations.